The Biology of
Success

The Biology of Success

Robert Arnot, M.D.

Little, Brown and Company
Boston • New York • London

First Edition

"A Morningness-Eveningness Questionnaire" from "A Self-Assessment Questionnaire to Determine Morningness-Eveningness in Human Circadian Rhythms" by J. A. Holmes and O. Öetberg originally published in *International Journal of Chronobiology*, vol. 4, pp. 97–110. Permission granted by Gordon and Breach Publishers.

Anxiety and depression quizzes from PRIME-MD Patient Health Questionnaire®, developed by Dr. Robert L. Spitzer, Dr. Janet B. W. Williams, Dr. Kurt Kroenke, and colleagues. PRIME-MD® is a trademark of Pfizer Inc. Copyright © 1999 Pfizer Inc. All rights reserved. Reproduced with permission.

Brian type survey from Jonathan P. Niednagel's book, *Your Key to Sports Success*.

Kay Foster-Powell's and Janette Brand-Miller's glycemic index tables adapted with permission from the *American Journal of Clinical Nutrition* 62 (1995): 871–935.

Library of Congress Cataloging-in-Publication Data
Arnot, Robert Burns.
    The biology of success / by Robert Arnot. — 1st ed.
        p.   cm.
    Includes index.
    ISBN 0-316-05161-6
    1. Mental health.   2. Success.   3. Self-management (Psychology)   I. Title.
RA790.5.A76   2000   99-36050

10 9 8 7 6 5 4 3 2 1

MV-NY

Text design by Joyce C. Weston
Printed in the United States of America

To my father, who has long shown
that honesty, integrity, and hard work
are the keys to success

Contents

Acknowledgments

I'd like to thank the following individuals who gave generously of their time to the undertaking of this book:

Kathryn Alexander, composer and Professor of Music Composition at Yale University.

F. Lee Bailey, trial lawyer.

Judith Ben Hurley, herb specialist, journalist, and author of *The Good Herb* and *Healing Secrets of the Seasons.*

Herbert Benson, M.D., Associate Professor of Medicine at Harvard Medical School, and author of *The Relaxation Response, Beyond the Relaxation Response,* and *Timeless Healing.*

Steven Blair, P.E.D., Director of Research at the Cooper Institute for Aerobic Research in Dallas, Texas.

Kenneth Blum, Ph.D., Research Professor in the Department of Biological Sciences at the University of North Texas, and Scientific Director of Path Medical Foundation in New York.

William F. Buckley Jr., author and journalist.

Robert Cialdini, Ph.D., Professor of Psychology at Arizona State University in Tempe, and author of *Influence: The Psychology of Persuasion.*

David Costill, Professor Emeritus of Exercise Physiology at Ball State University in Muncie, Indiana.

Richard Davidson, Ph.D., Professor of Psychology and Psychiatry at the University of Wisconsin–Madison.

Michael DeBakey, M.D., cardiovascular surgeon, Houston, Texas.

Ed Diener, Ph.D., the University of Illinois, Champaign–Urbana.

Derk-Jan Dijk, Ph.D., Assistant Professor of Medicine at Harvard Medical School.

Sheryl Dileo, Ph.D., MT-BC, Professor of Music Therapy, Temple University.

Andrea Dunn, Ph.D., Associate Director of the Division of Epidemiology and Clinical Applications at the Cooper Institute for Aerobics Research, Dallas, Texas.

Alan Flusser, clothes designer and author of *Style and the Man, Clothes and the Man,* and *Shopping around the World.*

John Forcy, M.D., Director of the Behavioral Medicine Research Center at Baylor College of Medicine in Houston, Texas.

Ellen Frank, M.D., of the University of Pittsburgh Medical Center's Western Psychiatric Institute and Clinic (WPIC).

Allan Geliebter, M.D., of the Obesity Research Center at St. Luke's–Roosevelt Hospital Center in New York.

William Glasser, M.D., founder and president of the William Glasser Institute in California, and author of *Choice Theory, A New Psychology of Personal Freedom* and *The Language of Choice Theory.*

Scott J. Goldsmith, M.D., Clinical Assistant Professor of Psychiatry at the Weill Medical College of Cornell University.

Harold Guskin, acting coach, New York.

Richard J. Haier, M.D., Department of Pediatrics at the University of California at Irvine.

Yuri Hanin, Ph.D., Professor and Senior Researcher at the Research Institute for Olympic Sports in Finland.

Joseph R. Hibbeln, M.D., National Institute on Alcohol Abuse and Alcoholism, one of the National Institutes of Health.

David Hircock, Director of the Aveda Aromatherapy Academy, and member of the Royal Pharmaceutical Society and the National Institute of Medical Herbalists.

Jim Horne, Director of the Sleep Research Laboratory Department of Human Sciences at Loughborough University, England, and coauthor of "A Self-Assessment Questionnaire to Determine Morningness-Eveningness in Human Circadian Rhythms."

Robert Jourdain, composer and author of *Music, the Brain, and Ecstasy.*

Jeffrey Kaye, M.D., the Oregon Health Sciences University in Portland, Oregon.

Father Thomas Keating, of St. Benedict's Monastery in Snowmass, Colorado, and author of *Open Mind Open Heart* and *Invitation to Love.*

Susan Knasko, M.D., the University of Pennsylvania.

Harold G. Koenig, M.D., Director of Duke University's Center for the Study of Religion/Spirituality and Health.

Daniel F. Kripke, M.D., Chronobiologist at the University of California at San Diego.

David Larson, M.D., President of the National Institute for Healthcare Research and adjunct Professor of Psychiatry at Duke Medical Center and Northwestern Medical School.

Joseph LeDoux, Ph.D., Professor of Psychology and Neuroscience at New York University, and author of *The Emotional Brain.*

James Loehr, Ed.D., of LGE Performance Systems Inc.

Dale A. Matthews, M.D., Associate Professor of Medicine at Georgetown University School of Medicine and author of *The Faith Factor.*

James Matthews, M.D., Professor of Psychology and Neuroscience at New York University.

Charles McCormack, President, Save the Children, USA.

Mark H. McCormack, pioneer in the business of athlete representation, and founder of International Management Group.

Emmanuel Mignot, M.D.–Ph.D., Director of the Center for Narcolepsy at Stanford University.

Timothy Monk, Ph.D., Professor of Psychiatry at the University of Pittsburgh.

Martin Moore-Ede, M.D.–Ph.D., founder and CEO of Circadian Technologies, Inc., the leading research and consulting firm helping companies and their employees work and live safely and productively in today's twenty-four-hour society.

William Morgan, Ed.D., Professor in the Department of Kinesiology at the University of Wisconsin–Madison.

Ralph Morris, Ph.D., Professor of Pharmacology at the College of Pharmacy at the University of Illinois.

Tom Murphy, Chairman of the Board of Save the Children, and longtime Chairman of the ABC Television Network.

Jonathan Niednagel, Ph.D., Director of the Brain Type Institute in California and author of *Your Key to Sports Success* and *Get the Most Out of Life with Your Inborn Brain Type.*

Dean Ornish, M.D., preventive medicine pioneer.

O. Ostberg of the Department of Occupational Health in Sweden, and coauthor of "A Self-Assessment Questionnaire to Determine Morningness-Eveningness in Human Circadian Rhythms."

Father M. Basil Pennington, of St. Joseph's Abbey in Spenser, Massachusetts, and author of *Centering Prayer.*

Leonard W. Poon, Ph.D., Professor of Psychology and Director of the Gerontology Center at the University of Georgia.

Christina Puchalski, M.D., Assistant Professor and Director of Clinical Research at the Center to Improve Care of the Dying at George Washington University School of Medicine, and Director of Education at the National Institute for Healthcare Research.

John J. Ratey, M.D., Assistant Clinical Professor of Psychiatry at Harvard Medical School.

Frances Rauscher, Ph.D., Assistant Professor of Cognitive Development at the University of California, Irvine.

Geshe Michael Roach, the Asian Classics Institute in New York.

Ellen Rosand, Ph.D., Professor of Music at Yale University.

Peter Salovey, Ph.D., Professor of Psychology and Epidemiology and Public Health at Yale University.

Ramon Satyendra, Ph.D., Associate Professor of Music at Yale University, and editor of *The Journal of Music Theory.*

Michael A. Schmidt, Ph.D., author of *Smart Fats* and Visiting Professor of Applied Biochemistry and Clinical Nutrition at Northwestern College.

Paul Schwartz of Sphere One Inc.

Martin Seligman, Ph.D., Professor of Psychology at the University of Pennsylvania and author of *Learned Optimism.*

Fran Shea, Acting President of E! Entertainment.

John Silber, Ph.D., Chancellor and former President of Boston University.

Robert Singer, Ph.D., Chairman of the Department of Exercise and Sport Sciences at the University of Florida.

Michael Smolensky, Ph.D., of the University of Texas School of Public Health.

David Spiegel, M.D., Director of the Psychosocial Treatment Laboratory at Stanford University School of Medicine.

Robert L. Spitzer, M.D., Professor of Psychiatry and Chief of Biometrics Research at the New York State Psychiatric Institute.

Andrew Stoll, M.D., of McLean Hospital and Harvard Medical School.

Michael Terman, Ph.D., Professor of Clinical Psychology in Psychiatry at Columbia University and Director of the Winter Depression Program at Columbia-Presbyterian Medical Center.

Susan Vaughan, M.D., Professor of Psychiatry at Columbia University College of Physicians and Surgeons, and author of *The Talking Cure.*

Alexander Vuckovic, M.D., psychiatrist at McLean Hospital in Belmont, Massachusetts, and Instructor in Psychiatry at Harvard Medical School.

Richard Webster, feng shui expert and author of *Feng Shui for Beginners, 101 Feng Shui Tips for the Home,* and *Feng Shui in the Workplace*

Michael Wenger, Dean of Buddhist Studies at the San Francisco Zen Center.

Tom West, Director of the Dyslexic Association and author of *In the Mind's Eye.*

Linda S. Wilson, Ph.D., President Emerita of Radcliffe College.

Judith J. Wurtman, Ph.D., Director of TRIAD Weight Management Center, McLean Hospital, an affiliate of Harvard Medical School.

Richard Wurtman, Ph.D., of the Massachusetts Institute of Technology.

David Wyon, Ph.D., of Johnson Controls.

Special Thanks to:

Rima Canaan for her diligence and keen intellectual insight and the months of hard work it took to complete *The Biology of Success.*

Laurence Kirshbaum, Chairman, Time Warner Books, for his wonderful spirit and tremendous backing.

Sarah Crichton, Publisher, Little, Brown, for her tremendous support and great good cheer.

Bill Phillips, my editor at Little, Brown, for his unflagging enthusiasm, tireless effort, and for so readily adapting the principles of this book into his own life.

Simon and Dan Green, my literary agents, for their decade-long support of my writing career.

Introduction

Life's biggest winners all exhibit tremendous, persistent positive mental energy. Whether in medicine, technology, government, and education, or in business, or in music and the arts, or in sports, winners have an energy that allows them to rise above the mundane, cut through the red tape, and experience the flashes of brilliance necessary to win in today's fiercely competitive world. We all know at least one such winner and have read about many more who seem naturally blessed with the qualities that allow them to bound through life with great zest. At times, as many of us struggle to get through the day, we look with envy on those rare individuals who seem to have limitless enthusiasm and who seem to accomplish so much more than we do. It must be in the genes or the luck of the draw, we think, wishing we could be so blessed. We look to IQ and other tests to validate our suspicion that success must quite simply be a matter of biological destiny. But history books and popular biographies are filled with the stories of those who succeeded despite performing miserably on standardized tests, failing in school, and somehow missing the other popular predictors of success. Why? Success is driven by positive mental energy and positive thought. Linda S. Wilson, President Emerita of Radcliffe College, says: "Positive thinking has an incredible effect on people and it unleashes creativity." The good news is that you too can create in yourself the bright moods, mental energy, and positive patterns of thought that underlie the accomplishments of our highest achievers.

But how many times have you tried? How many times have you started the day with good intentions, eager to do better, be more efficient, even humming the tune to the U.S. Army's jingle "Be all that you can be"? Yet as the day progressed your energy fell and your resolve waned. You bought organizers, little agenda books, filled notebooks with detailed schedules and lofty goals, but couldn't find the get-up-and-go. You read a pile of self-help books, but found them too vague and abstract. What's missing? Quite simply, the know-how to *create* and *manage* the mental energy required to accomplish great things.

What are those great things? What is success? I asked hundreds of experts, colleagues, and friends to define success. Most pointed out that money, title, and position were not the only answers. Success can be influencing and educating a hundred children a year, answered my friend Rick Grogan, a world-class oarsman and successful entrepreneur who expresses his greatest admiration for teachers. Raising wonderful, ethical, and responsible children answered my wife and my mother. For Charles McCormack, President of Save the Children, success is substantially improving the lives of children around the world through education, health care, and immunizations, and securing the children a future by providing work opportunities for their parents. For Mrs. Sadako Ogato, UN High Commissioner for Refugees, it's protecting the lives of 28 million refugees around the world on any given day. For Jack Welch, Chairman of General Electric, success means, in part, creating a great place to work and some of the greatest stock value in history.

Success is a scary word to many of us because we feel it has eluded us. We confuse fame and fortune with true success. Dr. Jim Loehr, a world-class sports psychologist who works forming champion athletes, gives this explanation: "Success comes from identifying an internal need or deficiency that motivates you, setting high goals, and connecting with an activity that fulfills that need." Some fulfill that internal need by helping people, others by becoming "king of the world," like *Titanic* director James Cameron, still others by amassing enormous amounts of money.

The Road Map

Think of the steps in this book as building a fire within. Here's why. You can't just throw three big oak logs and a match into a fireplace and expect a blazing fire. You've got to start with paper, kindling from smaller, softer woods, the right draft. So too with creating a fire within yourself. It is the foundation that makes the fire burn at all. That foundation is positive mental energy. This book will help you build a solid, roaring, long-lived fire that will allow you to thrive in the most adverse of situations. Here's how:

Part One: Create Mental Energy

Mental energy is both the currency of success and its most basic biological underpinning. You can think of this first section as building mental capital . . . capital you will want to preserve and increase with each passing day.

In each step of Part One, you'll find both strategic and tactical uses of the most highly effective means of creating mental energy. By strategic, I mean that employing these measures on a day-to-day basis will lift your overall long-term level of mental energy. By tactical, I mean that using these measures on a particular day will boost your mental energy for that day. Over the last fifteen years of reporting on advances in personal health and fitness, I've had a chance to search far and wide for what really works. Much of what you'll find in this book is the very best I've uncovered during those years of research and personal experimentation.

As you read Part One, you'll find yourself automatically incorporating many of the suggestions into your life. By the time you've reached the end, I hope you'll already feel consistently better than you've ever felt before. However, to be certain that you are reaping the full benefits of these guidelines, and to help you perform at your best every day, I have included at the end of Part One two helpful chapters: "Plan the Biologically Successful Day," a practical, sample daily guide that contains much of what you have learned in Part One; and a problem-solving or troubleshooting section.

Part Two: Create Positive Thought

Part Two will teach you how to create a positive pattern of thought. There is the tantalizing prospect that by establishing new patterns of thought, you're fundamentally changing the way your brain works so that you can undertake more ambitious and challenging goals.

The 1990s have been called "the decade of the brain," and indeed some of the most stunning scientific advances at the tail end of the twentieth century are in brain research. Researchers are developing the early tools to diagnose the inner workings of moods, emotions, and thought as these occur in the brain, so we can study more closely how to manipulate them. Genes for anxiety and even thrill seeking have been tentatively identified. Scientists can now peer into the living human brain with a PET scan, a sophisticated device that shows how active specific parts of the brain are. Mirroring the colors of the rainbow from darkest blue to brightest white, PET scans show the great excitement and activity in the brain. When centers of the brain come to life, the more active they are, the brighter the colors on the PET scan. Richard Davidson, Ph.D., Professor of Psychology and Psychiatry at the University of Wisconsin–Madison, found that the left prefrontal cortex of the brain is linked to positive thought and emotion. Individuals with increased left prefrontal cortex activity are happier and more positive and are able to turn off negative emotion. By contrast, subjects with increased right-sided anterior activation show an increased vulnerability to negative emotions, bad moods, and the psychopathology associated with withdrawal. Often they demonstrate negative affect, fear, and disgust, and are perhaps predisposed to certain phobias.

You can win and win big only by driving certain parts of your brain to fulfill their greatest potential. Part Two will help get you there using the most engaging and innovative techniques from learned optimism to emotional broadcasting. Several chapters have self-tests from which you can learn how to succeed based on your own personality and strengths. By the end of Part Two, you'll understand yourself better and be better able to channel your energy and enthusiasm in the directions that will maximize your success.

When Leonardo da Vinci first envisioned flight, it was an image of a single man flying in the most rudimentary frame with wings. Look at the wildest predictions of the previous centuries and you will notice that they did not even faintly foreshadow the vast advances made in flight during the twentieth century. Even the most forward-looking visionaries of their day did not envision jumbo jets, super-sonic aircraft, and space shuttles, nor the dizzying changes these aircraft would have on global economies and the movement of people and goods.

My friend Austin Hearst lives by the adage that "chance favors the prepared." Any number of life's most successful people just happened to be at the right place at the right time with the right attitude and the right preparation. This book will help you with that preparation by giving you the mental energy and winning attitude you'll need. Look at any person we consider successful today and what you see is seemingly boundless energy. From presidents and executives to headmistresses to singers and great authors, you see energy in motion. They don't drag through the day, they race through it. Not only can you be a success, but you should. You owe it to yourself, your family, and your friends.

This book will teach you how to harness the enormous mental energy and create the positive thought patterns necessary for success. The breakthrough I hope to impart to you is the sense of control you have over your own destiny, the power to create within yourself the biological underpinnings of success, in short . . . the Biology of Success.

PART ONE

Create Mental Energy

Build Mental Capital

Mental energy is the basic foundation of success. Look at corporate titans such as Michael Eisner, Martha Stewart, and Jack Welch, or world leaders such as Nelson Mandela, Tony Blair, and Margaret Thatcher, or super moms from Maria Von Trapp to Barbara Bush. High mental energy is what they all have or had in common. Mental energy is the brain's power supply — the more power you have, the longer and harder you can work. Compare your work output the morning after taking a red-eye to that after a refreshing night's sleep. It's brain energy that makes the difference.

> **CONVENTIONAL WISDOM:** Success is in the genes.
>
> **THE BIOLOGY OF SUCCESS:** Mental energy fuels success.

Affect

When you meet many successful people, it's not their actual brain energy that first strikes you, it's their affect. Affect is a more precise, medical term for mood. Most successful people have a high positive affect most of the time; not that they don't get cross, angry, and even down, but their predominant affect is positive.

A landmark paper published in 1985 by David Watson and Auke Tellegen concluded that most mood variations can be explained by just two factors: positive affect and negative affect.* Positive affect is

---

*D. Watson and A. Tellegen, "Toward a Consensual Structure of Mood," *Psychological Bulletin* 98 (1985): 219–235.

associated with enthusiasm, activity, strength, and elation; it's the opposite of dull, sluggish, or sleepy. Negative affect is associated with feelings such as nervousness, fear, distress, scorn, and hostility; it's the opposite of being calm or relaxed. Positive affect encompasses feelings relating to energy; negative affect encompasses feelings relating to tension.

A highly positive affect acts as the energizer needed to supercharge our thought processes. Ed Diener, Ph.D., of the University of Illinois, Champaign–Urbana, reports that it is positive affect that "motivates human sociability, exploration, and creativity." At work, you will be far more productive and much more likely to be helpful if you are in a positive mood. In short, good and bad moods determine your pattern of thought. "A negative mood *generates* sadness, irritability, guilt, and a negative, self-critical, and pessimistic thought pattern," says Dr. Diener.

Understanding positive and negative affect is absolutely critical to goal-setting. If goals require a great deal of energy and you think about them while in a low-energy mood, you may get discouraged and feel you can't achieve them, and as a result you'll set lower goals for yourself than you should. Robert E. Thayer, Ph.D., professor of psychology at California State University, Long Beach, writes in his excellent book *The Origin of Everday Moods,* "Your current energy level is incorrectly influencing your judgments about your ability to muster enough energy and commitment for the future task."* In other words, be aware that how you feel has a direct impact on your thinking processes. When we set standards for ourselves they seem objective, but standards and goal-setting are totally subjective and personal.

To be a success, you should set goals only when your mood and energy levels are elevated. Be aware, though, that if you set your goals at a one-time high (for example, when you just won the lottery), you may not be able to reach those goals because you'll not be able to find again the same high-energy and high-mood state. Using

---

*Robert E. Thayer, Ph.D., *The Origin of Everyday Moods* (New York: Oxford University Press, 1996), p. 20.

The Biology of Success, you will want to concentrate on bringing your overall affect and energy to a higher overall level *before* you set goals that dreams are made of . . . and then maintaining that energy to carry out your goals.

The Mood Thermostat

The brain's affect ranges from very low to very high. The right genes bless some of us with a high setting and a lifetime of happiness. Others among us are cursed with a low setting and years of bleak moods and dark thoughts. Although we talk about a wide range of emotions from happy and joyful to sad, angry, and outright hostile, for the purposes of thinking positively we are simply interested in whether our affect is positive or negative. The great good news is that you can create more mental energy, much like turning up a thermostat, only it is your brain energy levels that you arc readjusting to a higher setting.

This "mood thermostat" is located deep within the brain in a structure called the amygdala. Using brain scans, scientists can now peer into the amygdala and see in three-dimensional color its degree of activity. The relationship to mood is inverse: the lower the activity of the amygdala, the higher your mood.

A note of caution: Be aware of what I call the stepladder effect. In modern-day America, our national mood is one of anxiety, even mild depression. This is protective. When bad things happen, there is not far to fall. As your mental energy and mood rise, however, you'll find that it is as if you are on an unsteady stepladder. Sure you feel terrific, but you're afraid of falling should bad things happen. You may even start to look down in terror at how far you now have to fall. To build resilience against the stepladder effect, you need to immunize yourself with the spirit of optimism, which is discussed in the chapter "Be an Optimist" in Part Two. Life's biggest winners get knocked down again and again, but they fundamentally believe they can win; when adverse events plunge them into momentary despair or gloom, they just as quickly pull themselves back together and regain their positive affect and mental energy.

Where Is Your Thermostat Set?

Brain scanning is not routinely available for the diagnosis of low mood, but excellent self-tests are. The following self-test will help you determine where on the scale of sadness to happiness your mood "thermostat" is fixed. Once you complete the self-test, carefully read the "Diagnosis" section following it.

SELF-TEST

Devised by Robert L. Spitzer, M.D., Chief of Biometric Research at the New York State Psychiatric Institute, the PRIME-MD™ test can be completed without the help of a doctor. Dr. Spitzer has graciously allowed me to use his test in this book.

Question: Over the last two weeks, how often have you been bothered by the following?

Please answer

    A. NOT AT ALL

    B. SEVERAL DAYS

    C. MORE THAN HALF THE DAYS

    D. NEARLY EVERY DAY

If you're not certain, keep a calendar for the next two weeks and mark how many days you suffer from the following symptoms.

_____ 1. Little interest or pleasure in doing things?

_____ 2. Feeling down, depressed, or hopeless?

_____ 3. Trouble falling or staying asleep, or sleeping too much?

_____ 4. Feeling tired or having little energy?

_____ 5. Poor appetite or overeating?

_____ 6. Feeling bad about yourself — that you are a failure or have let yourself or your family down?

_____ 7. Trouble concentrating on things, such as reading the newspaper or watching television?

_____ 8. Moving or speaking so slowly that other people could have
       noticed? Or the opposite — being so fidgety or restless
       that you are moving around a lot more than usual?
_____ 9. In the last two weeks, have you had thoughts that
       you would be better off dead or of hurting yourself in
       some way?

DIAGNOSIS

- If you answered yes to question 9, you should immediately seek the assistance of a highly skilled psychiatrist. The psychiatrist can examine you more thoroughly to determine if you are truly suicidal or homicidal.

- If you answered question 1 or 2 with NEARLY EVERY DAY and five or more of questions 2 through 8 with NEARLY EVERY DAY, you are probably suffering from a major depression. If you are surprised to find yourself suffering from a major depression, remember the American Medical Association reports that most people with clinical depression are either undiagnosed or misdiagnosed. In fact, 20 percent of the population now suffers from depression, and that number is likely to grow. Tragically, half of those who have been depressed for twenty or more years have never taken an antidepressant. You will want to seek professional help and discuss with your doctor the benefits of talk therapy and drug therapy.

- If you answered SEVERAL DAYS to just two or more of the above questions, you suffer a low affect. In your current state, you'll have a hard time thinking positively without resetting your mood. John J. Ratey, M.D., Assistant Clinical Professor of Psychiatry at Harvard Medical School, has coined the phrase "shadow depression" to mean that you have fewer than the necessary criteria to have an actual clinical depression but may still find real difficulty meeting life's challenges and blame yourself for social, academic, and professional failures.* Dr. Spitzer goes even further, saying

---

*See John J. Ratey, M.D., and Catherine Johnson, Ph.D., *Shadow Syndromes* (New York: Pantheon Press, 1997).

that depression occurs along a spectrum, very much like an elevated cholesterol count or high blood pressure. Just because the elevation is mild does not mean it should not be treated.

• If you are not depressed but suffer from a low mood, you may still want to discuss drug or talk therapy with your doctor.

Whatever your test result, you'll find the guidelines in the following Steps of Part One quite helpful for raising your current mood state. If you're not clinically depressed, you can, without the help of drugs or a psychiatrist, start resetting your mood thermostat to a higher positive level. In Part One of this book, you'll learn how to increase positive mental energy with personal space, music, food, exercise, ritual, and other highly useful activities, all of which affect mental alertness.

Step 1: Activate the Alertness Triggers

——— |||||| ———

Ever roll into work on Monday morning feeling as if you've flown in from Hong Kong when you've only taken in the commuter train from Darien . . . your energy is sapped, concentration shot, and motivation minimal? The surprise is that you *are* suffering from jet lag, only it resulted not from the train ride but from poor management of your brain's biological clock, which acts, in part, as a pacemaker for mental energy. We all mismanage this pacemaker at times, and the result can be huge losses of productivity and creativity in the American workplace. Mismanagement of our pacemakers may also result in car wrecks or major airline disasters or tragic accidents such as Three Mile Island and Chernobyl.

> **CONVENTIONAL WISDOM:** I'm tough. I'll just push through the fog of mental fatigue.
> **THE BIOLOGY OF SUCCESS:** Manage your brain's pacemaker properly to create untold amounts of mental energy.

The Biology of Alertness

The major source of mental alertness comes from deep within the brain, from the master pacemaker called the endogenous circadian pacemaker or ECP. "Circadian" refers to a biological rhythm that repeats itself approximately every twenty-four hours; the word "circadian" comes from the Latin phrase "*circa* (about) *dies* (day)." The ECP is the central control center for sleep, alertness, and mental performance. The more common parlance for ECP is biological clock.

Why have a body clock? The human body is designed to be awake during the day and asleep at night, and the reason for this stems from prehistoric times: unlike other predatory animals, we have poor night vision, hearing, and smell, and so are highly vulnerable in the primitive forest at night. Our internal biological clock encourages us to retreat at night to the safety of our dwellings by virtually shutting down our operating systems and putting us to sleep. Although our needs today are very different from those of prehistoric times, our biological clocks remain imprinted with the time of prehistoric survival. In ten thousand years of recent human evolution, the circadian rhythm has not changed. During the morning hours, you'll probably find yourself alert and motivated to act. During certain nighttime hours and to a lesser extent during the late afternoon, you'll probably find most types of performance significantly impaired; manual dexterity, reaction time, mental arithmetic, and cognitive reasoning function measurably less well during these times.

Just as your alarm clock at the side of your bed cues you that it is time to get up, your biological clock is responsible for cueing you to certain times of the day — when to eat or when to sleep, for example. Our bodies display thousands of different rhythms, though we are conscious of only a few. Natural rhythms are found for almost every biological function, including sleep and wakefulness, body temperature, heart rate, blood pressure, blood sugar, and the production of hormones and digestive secretions. What you may not be aware of is that your moods are also monitored by this biological clock. Brain energy is no different from other natural rhythms, rising to its highest level or "mental prime time" in the first third of the day, around noon or 1 P.M., then dropping in the mid- to late afternoon, rising again to a subpeak in the early evening, and declining until sleep, then descending sharply in the wee hours until the lowest point, around 4 A.M. Energy is low at awakening, but is lowest just before bedtime.

As Dr. Timothy Monk of the University of Pittsburgh puts it, the biological clock is like the conductor of a symphony orchestra, directing temperature, hormones, blood pressure, and heart rate as he would different rhythms for different instruments of an orchestra.

If everything is going right, then you have one conductor beating one tempo and the orchestra plays together in harmony. However, say you fly to a different time zone. The first conductor disappears and a second conductor suddenly steps up and starts a different beat. Some instruments in the orchestra change right away; some take more time. The result is that you have lost the temporal harmony in your biological clock. This is called internal desynchronization and explains the feeling of malaise that sets in with jet lag. Our biological rhythms must be as finely tuned as a Formula One race car for maximum performance. When a race car is out of sync, fuel is poorly distributed, some cylinders are hotter than others, wheels aren't balanced, tire pressures are off, and steering is misaligned. Sure, the car runs, but it's not going to win any races.

The idea of a biological clock may sound like a lot of complicated neurobiology, but there is one key concept: light. Light synchronizes and sets our biological clock. Here's how.

In the retina there are light receptors that are connected to the biological clock or ECP through a neurological pathway. These light receptors in the retina send information about the time of day and the length of day to the biological clock, which in turn sends out dozens of specific commands to the body.

At the heart of your biological clock are two hormones: melatonin and cortisol. In the simplest sense, melatonin puts us to sleep and cortisol wakes us up.

In the evening, the pineal gland releases melatonin, which acts on our hypothalamus to make us sleepy. The faster melatonin is released or the more that is released, the faster you fall asleep. Younger people go to sleep faster and easier because they secrete more melatonin. During the day, melatonin is typically at a minimum, then it's released at bedtime and peaks in the middle of the night. Arbitrarily, if you go to sleep at 10 P.M. and wake at 6 A.M., around 1:30 A.M. or 2 A.M. melatonin will be at its peak and then it will taper off. By the time you rise at 6 A.M., melatonin is down to its minimum. Whatever precipitates the release of melatonin will facilitate going to sleep. A steady sleep pattern is critical to your circadian rhythm, because melatonin's release cycle does not shift easily. This failure to shift is the primary reason we suffer jet lag. The lag is in changing the time when melatonin is secreted.

Cortisol by contrast makes you more alert. Cortisol is the stress hormone. It gets switched on around 1 to 2 A.M. in anticipation of wakefulness. It is instrumental in waking up your body. Cortisol peaks around 9 to 11 in the morning and falls over the course of the day.

Many other hormones are also related to your biological clock. Thyroid hormone, for instance, is higher during the day than at night. This is important because thyroid hormone improves metabolism, mood, and activity. In fact, adding thyroid hormone to antidepressant medications can dramatically improve the effect of the medication, even in patients with normal thyroid functioning.

Mistiming any single hormone release can ruin your day. Now imagine having a dozen of them all out of whack. That leads to disruption of natural sleep/wake tendencies, desynchronization of daily body rhythms, and degeneration of sleep quality. These factors combine to reduce vigilance, seriously impair our judgment and decision-making ability, and destroy our overall efficiency and level of success. Pure misery is the result. To ensure daily performance and avoid sometimes catastrophic errors, you should become keenly attuned to your circadian rhythm and use understanding of your individual circadian rhythm to manage effectively alertness and fatigue.

Creating the Biology of Alertness

While your biological clock switches alertness on and off, you also have the power to enhance this alertness. You can learn to raise the valleys with the foods, light, exercise, music, and other brain-energy-elevating maneuvers contained in this book. All of these suggested maneuvers help to improve alertness by affecting one or more of the nine alertness switches proposed by Martin Moore-

Ede, M.D.–Ph.D., founder and CEO of Circadian Technologies, Inc., the leading research and consulting firm helping companies and their employees to work and live safely and productively in today's twenty-four-hour-a-day society (www.circadian.com).

1. *Interest, opportunity, and a sense of danger.* Nothing will pull you faster out of a drowsy state than the imminent threat of danger; and while I'm not advocating chasing danger, I am suggesting that you seek exciting pursuits that will activate this alertness switch. A stimulating job, for instance, can pull you into a greater state of alertness. When I asked Dr. Michael DeBakey, the ninety-year-old world-famous cardiac surgeon known as the Texas Tornado, how he still maintains a nineteen-hour day, he said: "If you are interested in what you do . . . and you're interested enough, the mental energy will come. It becomes a self-motivating factor." Attorney F. Lee Bailey agrees: "The stimulation inherent in exciting activity — animated cross examination, etc. — provides a kind of fuel (adrenaline, no doubt), which provides energy for both physical and intellectual feats."

2. *Environmental light.* Light adjusts the timing of your pacemaker or biological clock. The kind and quality of light you have makes a big difference in how you feel. Bright light tends to increase alertness, while dim light leads to drowsiness. You have heard about light therapy's positive effect in treating winter depression (known as Seasonal Affective Disorder or SAD); now light therapy is something all of us can use to regulate better our pacemaker. Step 2, "Build Creative Space," has lots more on this.

3. *Sleep bank balance.* How long you have been awake and how much sleep you have had in recent days dramatically affects alertness levels. When sleep-deprived for several days, you build up a "sleep debt" that leads to a decrease in alertness. A long spell of sleep acts as a deposit and offsets your sleep debt. Sleep is good for mood, and lack of sleep is bad for mood. The key to starting each day on the right foot is to have a good night's sleep. Sounds obvious, but it makes a real world of difference. Nearly 100 million Americans have sleep problems that rob them of performance. The chapter at the

end of Part One, "Maximize Alertness," has a full set of great sleep-enhancing recommendations.

4. *Muscular activity.* Walking and stretching trigger the sympathetic nervous system that helps you keep alert. Sitting idle in a comfortable chair can make it hard to stay awake. Some executives stand at a podium-like desk to stay alert. The Step on exercise, "Get Breathless," has guidelines and a full description of beneficial activities.

5. *Ingested nutrients and chemicals.* Certain foods and substances, such as proteins or caffeine, temporarily increase alertness; others — for example, bananas, warm milk, or sleeping pills — induce sleep. Step 4, "Eat for Mental Energy," lays out which foods to eat for optimal performance and which to avoid.

6. *Temperature.* Cool, dry air, especially on your face, helps keep you alert, while heat and humidity make you drowsy. The Step "Build Creative Space" has a terrific section on controlling temperature.

7. *Sound.* Great music can increases alertness and productivity, while overhearing loud conversations or a honking horn can stress and distract you. The sound of rolling waves on the beach or the hum of white noise from a machine can lull you to sleep. The Step "Build Creative Space" will show you how to control sound in your environment so that you remain stimulated in a productive way; and Step 3, "Turn On the Tunes," will help you increase alertness with terrific music.

8. *Aroma.* Studies have found that some smells such as peppermint make people more alert. Other smells such as lavender have a sedative effect. Step 2, "Build Creative Space," has more on the power of aroma.

9. *Time of day on biological clock.* Finally, mood and alertness are hugely influenced by the actual time set on your biological clock. As your circadian clock approaches its lowest level of wakefulness, this is also when your mood levels reach their lowest values. That's why life can seem so bleak whenever you awaken in the wee

hours and start to worry. While it is certainly important to try to establish a steady good mood, it is equally important to understand that even an upbeat individual is not fully charged 100 percent of the time. There are natural ebbs and flows, natural ups and downs that occur with each twenty-four-hour cycle. There are also longer cycles — weekly and monthly as well as seasonal cycles. Understanding these natural patterns is the key to success, since by doing so you will know when you're most productive and when you should just kick back. Lots of us try to maintain a steady state of high mental energy all day long, ignoring the natural rhythms in our mood clock. It's actually reassuring to know that it's normal to feel down and depressed first thing in the morning; you should not, however, let that initial low mood color your entire day. Remind yourself that a half hour from now you'll be feeling a lot better. If you give in to the idea that you should feel like the sprightly man or woman in a breakfast-cereal commercial, then you will think there is something wrong with you, and that will ruin your attitude for the rest of the day.

These nine switches work together. Someone who works outside, constantly surrounded by changing scenery and noise, different temperatures and smells, may be more alert even if less focused than someone in a cubicle with the quiet hum of a computer, the constant temperature of a controlled environment, and the same four walls surrounding him or her. Turning off too many alertness switches leads to microsleep and automatic responses. Microsleeps are brief unintended episodes of loss of attention associated with blank stares, head snapping, prolonged eye closure, and so on, which may occur when you are fatigued but are trying to stay awake to perform a monotonous task such as driving a car or watching a computer screen. Such microsleeps are most likely to occur at certain times of the day — during predawn and midafternoon hours when the pacemaker generates a low amount of alertness.

Be aware of your mood and energy levels as each day progresses. Every day for two weeks keep a mood diary about how you feel at different times of the day. Record in two columns "mood" and "energy" and observe yourself several times at different set times each day. See if you can detect a pattern in your mood and behavior. Focus on your energy highs and lows. Try to discern differences as well as similarities in your day-to-day behavior and feelings. You will find that different activities have vastly different effects, depending on when you undertake them. For instance, eating a carbohydrate for lunch will make you sleepy and groggy during the afternoon, while the same carbos late in the afternoon might help cut tension. Exercise in the morning will help build a morning energy peak but may leave you more tired later in the day, while exercise in the late afternoon will elevate your mood at the time of day when mood is near its lowest.

Focus

There's little sense in having huge amounts of mental energy if you can't focus it tightly like a laser, if you scatter it around through anxiety or tension, or too many energy-draining, unimportant tasks. In any performance-oriented task, performance increases as mental energy and motivation increase.

Psychologist Robert E. Thayer, Ph.D., explains that from a practical standpoint, what we ideally want for high performance is a state of energetic calm, when mental energy is high, but tension, anxiety, and restlessness are not out of control.* With increasing tension and anxiety, performance sharply drops. You want to keep your anxiety and tension low enough and energy high enough to truly focus like a laser. Step 9, "Preserve Mental Capital," contains the most powerful guidelines on how to stay focused by avoiding the big killers of mental energy and alertness.

---

*See Robert E. Thayer, Ph.D., *The Origin of Everyday Moods* (New York: Oxford University Press, 1996).

Step 2: Build Creative Space

Enter the inner sanctum of one of the nation's most successful CEOs. You'll notice dark mahogany paneling, beautiful paintings, and hushed tones. The lighting is quiet. There is even a smell of success. Follow that same CEO to the corporate aircraft, a gleaming $37 million Grumman Gulfstream V or Boeing Business Jet. The inside of the aircraft, worth a cool $3 million, feels like a tranquilizer: beautiful flowers, great smells, quiet elegance. Even in the air, there is never an unpleasant moment. Is this all spoiled self-indulgence? Hardly. This is the carefully constructed environment of success. *Fortune* 500 companies have spent millions studying the effect of environment on their workers and trying to invent and provide the most effective workplace possible. The fact that life for those at the top includes limos, private jets, and fresh flowers is not an accident; they keep the boss happy but also keep her mood up, so she can be positive and perform.

So you may say, "Sure, Doctor Bob, give me a $37 million jet and I promise to be happy too!" But happiness often has less to do with money than with a comfortable and rewarding work environment. I've been impressed that in even the poorest of circumstances, people create around them organization, style, and an environment that leads to financial prosperity and outstanding success. Mother Teresa created one of the world's greatest charities out of very modest, basic, but well-organized surroundings. William F. Buckley chooses to work in a converted three-car garage. "Everything I need is here. There is also an adjacent library, a converted toolshed. I have a direct line to my office in New York." He uses a computer to conserve space and suggests, "Use computer technology, the greatest space saver in history." You don't have to have an expensive environment, but you do need a clean, creativity-enhancing environment to propel you toward the outer limits of success. Tom Murphy was Chairman of Cap Cities/ABC for years; he says, "Good light is the most important thing for me. That's all I need — good light and a desk and phone."

> **CONVENTIONAL WISDOM:** Tough guys can work anywhere.
> **THE BIOLOGY OF SUCCESS:** The right space paves the road to success.

Environmental psychologists study every facet of human performance and create an environment to enhance it. In today's frantic world we can't always be in a space of our choosing. Outside forces can have tremendous impact on our ability to create positive mental energy. Just like the CEO in his jet, you'll want to build your own physical and psychological work "cocoon." General Patton brought his best linen, crystal, and china to war. You'll want to create a personal space you feel confident in, then bring that confidence and sense of calm out into the world.

The Biology of Your Personal Environment

Johnson Controls is the world's largest facility management company, managing everything from finances to fire concerns, security, heating, cooling, water, and sewage. Johnson Controls oversees 2,000 hospitals, 4,000 school districts, and one billion square feet of other people's office space. The company created the very first individual heating controls for hotel rooms more than one hundred years ago. David Wyon, Ph.D., of Johnson Controls, is a specialist in indoor environmental quality. He says the several main considerations for creating an environment conducive to success are the same for a large, multinational company as they are for you; in order of importance, these four crucial categories are TEMPERATURE, AIR QUALITY, LIGHTING, and ACOUSTICS. To help you create maximum energy levels, I'm adding a fifth and sixth category: AROMA and SPACE DESIGN. Whereas the first five categories are grounded in hard science, the sixth, space design, draws from a practice usually foreign to us here in the West — the ancient Chinese art of feng shui. For us Westerners, feng shui in its details presents a foreign, inaccessible-seeming worldview; but I have found the basic principles of feng shui to transform dramatically my work space into an area of increased productivity, and I am including in my discussion only the general directives that I found most effective.

Temperature

Have you ever heard the expression "It's too hot to think"? Well, this is not just an empty phrase. Temperature tops the list of complaints that people have about their work environment. No wonder. Thermal variations have the biggest influence on mental and manual performance. Here are the key factors you'll want to control.

Air temperature

Air temperature is the most critical element in thermal balance. In the United States, the optimum temperature for mental work is 70°F. Not everyone shares the same optimal temperature level. We call some people "hot-blooded" if they don't ever seem to get cold. Others are called "cold-blooded" because they are always putting on sweaters and coats. There is also a wider range for factory workers, depending on the climate they live in. In Europe, optimal temperature for factory work is 64°F. In South Africa, people are heat acclimatized to work best at 86°F; if temperatures cool below that, work performance suffers. Some experts believe that intellectual thought is greatly hampered when the temperature is much more than 70°F. Mental performance, rule-based logical thinking, for example, can be reduced by 30 percent at temperatures not even warm enough to cause sweating. The way heat stress affects mental performance is by altering levels of arousal in the brain. Mathematical tasks require high arousal, but heat makes for low arousal . . . the languid behavior we see at high noon in the tropics. While I was reporting on the recent famine in Sudan and the flare-up in the Sudanese civil war, temperatures were well over 100°F every day. There was no respite in air-conditioned cars or buildings. The heat made it so hard to think that it took an hour to do what would ordinarily take four minutes in a nicely air-conditioned building at home. As heat fatigue increases during the day, your alertness falls. Temperatures below optimum have no adverse effects on mental performance but do show effects on manual performance — in the cold, you first lose fingertip-movement speed, then fingertip sensitivity, then muscular strength. The best solution is to regulate individually your own optimal work temperature. In my home office I have an air conditioner that I use year-round to make sure that it's cool enough to think. Says William F. Buckley, "I would suffer if I didn't have an air conditioner."

Radiant temperature

You may have a perfectly controlled average room temperature, but could find yourself uncomfortable because of cold from a window or broiling heat from a steaming radiator. If you can't control your office temperature, you can customize your own office by changing radiant heat, using a heater for your feet, as an example. Dr. Wyon has developed an apparatus called a "Climadesk," which can warm thighs while keeping the face cool by providing optional thermal radiation to the lower parts of the body and optionally increased air movement to the upper parts (since temperatures increase with height above the floor, a space heater would not be able to provide the combination of warm feet/cool air to breathe). Moreover, unlike a space heater, which would raise air temperature for everybody in the room, the "Climadesk" allows individuals in the same room to experience very different resultant temperatures by providing optionally different rates of cooling or heating. And finally, the "Climadesk" can deliver fresh air directly into the breathing zone. The "Climadesk" is widely available in Sweden, and may soon be used more in the U.S. You could add a foot heater and fan to your desk until yours arrives!

Air velocity

Air velocity is the speed at which air is moving around you and is important because it is one factor that controls the speed at which you lose heat — and if you lose heat too quickly you'll grow cold, whereas if you're not losing heat quickly enough you'll feel hot and sluggish. You can affect the air velocity in your room by opening or closing a window, or switching a fan on or off. This may seem obvious, but I've spent countless nonproductive hours trying to figure out why I was uncomfortable, what was wrong and how to fix it, when an easy answer would have been just to open or close a window. Since you may not have control over the temperature, changing radiant heat and air velocity are good alternatives.

Humidity

Relative humidity is the amount of humidity in the air compared to how much humidity the air will take. Air humidity is usually in the 20 percent to 60 percent range. In the winter, when heating and cold dry air from outdoors reduce the relative humidity indoors to uncomfortable levels, consider buying a humidifier. I've found that it makes a world of difference in work comfort and prevents the dried-out mucous membranes that lead to a stuffy nose in the winter. When humidity levels become suffocating in the summer, an air conditioner quickly lowers humidity levels. Under winter conditions, 30 percent humidity is most comfortable for most people, according to Dr. Wyon's studies. Under summer conditions, when people are more lightly dressed, 50 percent humidity is acceptable and comfortable. If you're sweating, however, whether in the winter or in the summer, every percent that you can lower the humidity will help you feel more comfortable, because it will increase the rate of evaporative heat loss.

Metabolic rate

The *Today* show studio is freezing cold to most people. But to the active, high-energy news anchors and guests who inhabit it, it's heaven, because they won't find themselves sweating under the hot lights. Metabolic rate dramatically changes what you require from a room. If you're just back from a workout, you'll want a lower temperature, lower humidity, and a good brisk fan. If you're sitting quietly reading for hours at a time, cold temperatures can be quite uncomfortable and distracting. So think about your metabolic rate, how physically active you'll be in your work space, and design a work space that can accommodate changing the heat and humidity as your metabolic rate changes.

Clothing

Years ago, you would plunk down several thousand dollars at a great Savile Row tailor. In return, you got a great English bespoke suit. But to create truly stunning works of art, English tailors used fabric of great depth — fabric that was often 14- or even 16-ounce cloth, contrasted to the 8-ounce cloth used by many top Italian designers. Then central heating and global warming arrived. Almost no one can wear these masterpieces to work any longer. They're just too warm. Armani suits have become a favorite because they're incredibly light and lack the thick insulated liners of the old English suit. Heat balance is dramatically affected by what you wear. There's even a science involved. In the field of textile science the term "clo" is used as the unit of clothing. Normal insulation is 1.0 clo, which for a man would correspond to a suit with shirt; 1.0 clo is what a man would wear to be comfortable indoors in the winter. Similarly, 0.5 clo means half of the insulation regarded as normal. In the summer, a woman can go down to 0.5 clo, and a man can go down to 0.7 clo, which would correspond to a very light suit and light shirt. Unless men wear short pants, they can't go down in clo quite as much as women. The highest comfortable indoor clo is 1.5, which corresponds to a sweater and suit. Around the office I usually wear a pair of khakis and a cotton shirt, both of which have a low clo. If you're too cold, you can then add a jacket or sweater to improve your work efficiency.

Although a plus-or-minus-10°F range satisfies 99 percent of us in our offices, don't just peg the thermometer at 70 degrees. Now that you know the six key factors for thermal balance, take all six factors into consideration. Understand that you have your unique "normal" temperature. You'll know when you've hit it, because you'll be neither hot nor cold. The technical name for this is "neutrality." Neutrality can change depending on your metabolism at any given moment — whether you're sitting, are moving around, or have just finished a workout. When the temperature rises above neutrality, your mental abilities deteriorate, and, as mentioned before, when the temperature sinks below neutrality, your physical abilities are impaired.

Air Quality

Indoor air quality is nearing an all-time low, and many of us are paying the price. Today an increasing number of people are allergic to particles in indoor air. Studies show that indoor overexposure to pollen, mold, household dust, and animal skin and hair does indeed increase allergies. Possible negative reactions can range from a mere sensitivity to a strong allergy. More and more people, especially children, are asthmatic . . . and sealed buildings lurk as the number one reason. In Scandinavia, where people have learned to seal buildings to save energy, respiratory problems are especially bad.

Indoor air quality is measured by the amount of carbon monoxide in the air. The more fresh air there is, the lower the level of carbon monoxide. In fresh air there's 600 ppm (parts per million) of carbon monoxide. When you reach 1,000 ppm of carbon monoxide, the air starts to become stuffy. The recommended amount of fresh air is a minimum 10 cubic feet per minute per person. In Norway, only when researchers increased fresh air in schools up to 20 cubic feet per minute per child, did they raise the air quality to an optimum level. And in classrooms where ventilation had been improved, children showed reduced symptoms of ill health and better performance of a simple task (simple reaction time). Yet every cubic foot of fresh air brought in from the outside costs a lot of money; and so efforts to save money exacerbate the allergy problem.

Here's what you can do. First, if you have a choice, work in a building in which you can open the windows. If you work in a sealed building, lobby to increase your individual allotment of fresh air to 20 cubic feet per minute. Can't fight city hall? Curiously, an office or bedroom can contain more allergens than are found outdoors. Buy an electrostatic air cleaner to remove indoor allergens. You can actually see cigarette smoke go into an electrostatic air cleaner, and it doesn't come back out. They are still expensive, but as the technology improves, the prices will go down.

Also consider an ionizer, which improves air quality in your indoor space. In the natural environment, there are more ions in cleaner air, and less ions in less clean air. Negative ions have a positive effect on mood by releasing more of the neurotransmitter serotonin — thunderstorms release negative ions, and notice how you feel better at the end of a thunderstorm. You can now buy inexpensive negative ion generators for your office. Sphere One makes a good ionizer for home use; check their Web site at www.sphereone.com, or call (212) 208-4438.

Light

We often underrate the sun's influence on our mood. Michael Terman, Ph.D., is a Professor of Clinical Psychology in Psychiatry at Columbia University and a specialist in light therapy. Dr. Terman points out that the sun, even when it just peeps over the horizon, is already much brighter than indoor light. At daybreak, with the first glimmer of light, we already measure 800 lux of light in the atmosphere. By contrast, indoors, we consider 500 lux of light sufficient — and that's optimistic; 500 or 600 lux is what you might measure in a well-designed draftsman's studio. So just imagine how little light your dim indoor work environment provides compared to the natural outdoors! In effect, in our apartments and offices, we're in the twilight all day long. The modern urban lifestyle that keeps us indoors imposes darkness to such an extent that many people can seem chronically light-deprived and exhibit what seems like depression or a seasonal affective disorder all the time.

In the United States, most offices use overhead light, so all employees receive the same amount of light. That's bad news for many, because different people need different amounts of light at different times of the day. As a flexible light solution for the office, buy yourself a desk light that you can control. Here's the kind and intensity of light you need.

Since room light rarely exceeds 600 lux, and since you need at least 1,000 lux to start reaping the biological benefits of light, consider installing a special lighting system. By "lighting system" I mean an apparatus (not just individual bulbs) that you buy in a store. When you buy a lighting apparatus, the bulbs are in a configuration in a system with the specific filtering and bulb placement that are critical design factors. Unless you are a lighting engineer, you would not know how to construct such a lighting system, and if you did, it would surely cost you more to do it yourself than to buy a ready-made apparatus.

Dr. Terman, who advocates use of a lighting system, recommends the Sphere One Lighting Apparatus. The bulbs installed in the Sphere One apparatus offer white illumination. Sphere One carefully screens its lighting systems for ultraviolet illumination and attenuates the blue range of light; the blue range of light is non-optimal for long-term exposure because blue photons are very energetic and bounce around the eyeball, creating a glare sensation that is very unpleasant at high intensity. In addition to offering the best short-wavelength attenuation available on the marketplace, Sphere One systems produce a softer sensation of light at higher intensities and have been tested in clinical trials, an important criterion to consider when choosing a system. Sphere One sells "Sphere Daylight 10,000," an apparatus that exposes you to 10,000 therapeutic lux when you sit at a certain distance from it — if you suffer from "winter blues" you'll want to consider buying this apparatus and you'll also want to turn to "Maximize Alertness: Problem Solving" at the end of Part One to learn in detail how to use light to combat "winter blahs." Sphere One also sells a deluxe model with different settings that allow you to switch the lux down during the day if you want to use the apparatus for desktop or change the lux again for the living room in the evening. You can order these systems by calling Sphere One at (212) 208–4438. Sphere One does have the advantage of solid scientific testing — its systems are somewhat expensive, nearly $500, but they're worth the investment if your work space is poorly lit or you suffer symptoms of winter depression.

Acoustics

Sound pollution is most annoying and distracting in the work environment. While you can turn your head and look away from a visual distraction, noise is far more invasive. Why? Noise demands a series of cognitive decisions that take us away from the task at hand. There are three steps in hearing noise: detect it, identify it, and interpret it. Only then can you suppress it. Distracting sounds undermine your concentration and allow your thoughts to drift. Many people are frustrated by the little noises that surround them — street traffic, the sound of someone pacing around on the floor above, noisy plumbing; but the worst distraction is the human voice, because we can't help but listen to people talking. For some people it can never be quiet enough. Even in the bucolic countryside bird cries or insect chirpings can be a distraction.

Rather than fall into the trap of looking everywhere for a place that is quiet enough, seize control of sound in your environment and neutralize it. When you create an ideal working space, don't let whatever random sound already populates your environment take over; create for yourself a kind of personal "soundscape." Many people use noise generators to blanket or cover distracting noise information so that they can concentrate on their work. If you're going to use a noise generator, Dr. David Wyon recommends a pink-noise generator. So-called white-noise generators do wipe out bad sounds but produce a high-frequency hiss. The human ear associates high frequency with danger, and low frequency with slow movement and soft impact. Pink-noise generators (called pink by analogy because red light has a lower frequency than blue light) have a lower frequency and attenuate the higher frequencies, resulting in a subjective impression that the noise is softer. All noise generators sold today are white noise, but David Wyon says you can easily create your own pink-noise generator. To create pink noise, buy an amplifier or a radio with a graphic equalizer (the cheaper the better since cheaper amplifiers produce more noise), turn down the treble to attenuate higher frequencies, and the remaining lower frequency hiss is pink noise! Self-contained stereo systems cost only several hundred dollars and also deliver terrific sound. The easiest approach I've found is using a fan or an air conditioner. I turn on an air conditioner, even in the winter, to kill outside noise.

Aroma

Researchers are exploring and discovering the benefits of aromatherapy for, among other things, insomnia, anxiety, weight loss, pain management, concentration problems, and heart ailments. Aromatherapy is taught at medical institutions throughout Germany and England; now the first postgraduate course is being offered in the United States at Purdue University. Throughout the United States, however, some medical fields already use aromatherapy as a complement, not an alternative, to other therapies. A study at the Old Manor Hospital in Salisbury, Britain, found that diffused lavender essential oil could successfully replace medication to relieve insomnia. A study at a New York hospital used the fragrance heliotropin (an aroma found in nature in vanilla and black pepper) during MRI (magnetic resonance imaging) procedures to reduce anxiety levels, and found that the group exposed to the aroma experienced 63 percent less anxiety than the control group that couldn't smell the fragrance. In another study, at the Royal Shrewsbury Hospital in Britain, aromatherapy oil (lavender, jasmine, and ylang ylang) was diffused throughout the coronary care ward, and results showed a 71 percent reduction in anxiety levels as opposed to a 25 percent reduction in anxiety for persons in the control portion of the trial. Psychiatrist and neurologist Dr. Alan Hirsch studied the effects of using special aroma cassettes (an aroma cassette is a plastic inhaler that holds an aroma on an absorbent pad, and by opening the top of the cassette you can easily smell the aroma) to assist people with weight loss, and found that during his six-month study, patients lost an average of thirty pounds; the most effective fragrances were the ones that the patients liked best. Further studies have shown that certain aromas increase work task performance. Rosemary helps improve concentration and aids in overcoming learning difficulties. In the workplace in Japan, lemon essence is often transmitted through the ventilation system to increase worker productivity. A study at the coronary unit of the Royal Sussex Hospital in Britain showed that aromatherapy combined with massage could help alleviate pain and reduce blood pressure and heart rate.

David Hircock, director of the Aveda Aromatherapy Academy and member of both the Royal Pharmaceutical Society and the National Institute of Medical Herbalists, has helped design an herbal medicine degree course. He explained to me how aromatherapy works.

There are two olfactory pathways for smells to reach the brain — a main and an accessory pathway.

The main pathway originates in the sensory neurons in the nose and ends in the main olfactory bulb. When we inhale through our noses, the smell stimulus goes directly to the creative, right side of the brain and to what is often called the limbic system or our "first" brain, our "emotional" brain. When smell stimulates the limbic system, it can stimulate hormone release.

The accessory pathway originates in sensory neurons located in the floor of the nasal cavity, and terminates in the accessory olfactory bulb. Recent studies indicate that the accessory olfactory pathway plays an important role in the recognition of odors associated with sexual behaviors.

Smell is our first sense — it's our chemical sense. Olfaction was important even when all organisms were a primordial stew; olfaction is originally one of the main senses of fish and bacteria. So powerful is our sense of smell that we can detect just one-millionth of one milligram of garlic molecules floating in the air. That's the equivalent of tasting a drop of vinegar in a swimming pool. And you can even tell where the odor is coming from because it reaches one nostril before the other.

Not only is smell our first sense, but it is also our most immediate sense, which is perhaps why fragrance-evoked memories are so strong. With sight, for example, light first has to go through the iris and retina on the way to the brain. Sight involves several electrical pathways, many synapses, before it is processed by the brain. Aroma, by contrast, takes a much more direct path to the brain, involves only a few synapses, and is almost instantaneously processed. In fact, olfaction is the sense physically closest to the limbic system, which includes the hippocampus (implicated in working memory and short-term memory) and the amygdala (responsible for emotions). A recent study indicates that only two synapses separate the olfactory nerve from the amygdala and only three synapses separate the olfactory nerve from the hippocampus.

How to apply aromatherapy

Using essential oils or the essence of plants, you can administer aromatherapy in a several ways. Always remember to dilute the essential oils. All essential-oil bottles have integral droppers, so it is easy to control the number of drops you use:

- Bath: This method is most effective with calming fragrances. Wait until the water has stopped running and the bath is full of warm water, then put 3–4 drops of essential oil in the water, swirl the water around, sit back, breathe in, and relax.

- Shower: This method is best for energizing fragrances. Drop two drops of essential oil on the shower floor in front of your feet, and then shower as usual. Note, however, that essential oils dissolve plastic, so if your shower is made of ceramic, you can put the essential oil drops directly on the ceramic, but if your shower is made of plastic, put the two oil drops on a small washcloth and leave the washcloth at your feet while you're showering.

- Massage: Mix 3–6 drops of essential oil in an ounce of massage-oil base, such as almond oil or grapeseed oil. Massage with the soothing massage oil.

- Diffuser: A diffuser, also called an "aroma-lamp," has a small dish on top and a candle underneath. Fill the dish with water, add to the water a few drops of essential oil, and light the candle. Sit back and smell the aroma. This is the best method for your office.

- Essential-oil candles: You can also buy and light these, but make sure they are natural essential-oil candles.

You can buy essential oils, massage-oil base, diffusers, and candles in most herb stores, health-food stores, department stores, and aromatherapy specialty stores.

Specific aromas for your mood

There are two key ways to drink in mood-changing aromas. The first is by using essential oils, which you can strategically place in your environment. The second is through juices and herbal teas.

ESSENTIAL OILS

Following are some of the most powerful mood-changing aromas listed in two categories: relaxants and energizers. Relaxants act on neuropeptides, causing a relaxation response, while energizers cause an instant energy boost. You can use drops of these oils in baths for relaxants, in showers for energizers, with massage-oil bases or diffusers, or you can buy candles containing these essential oils.

RELAXANTS

- Lavender
- Ylang ylang (ylang ylang is a tropical flower that grows in Malaysia and Indonesia)
- Rose
- Chamomile
- Geranium
- Sandalwood
- Frankincense
- Jasmine

ENERGIZERS

- Peppermint (Peppermint decreases your skin temperature, which indicates that the blood has gone from the skin to the brain and to muscles.)

- Citrus oils: lemon, lemongrass, mandarin orange

- Eucalyptus (Eucalyptus is good for combating fatigue, particularly fatigue relating to sinus or stuffiness. Candlemakers often use eucalyptus because of its energizing powers.)

- Rosemary (Rosemary is uplifting, energizing, and reported to be especially good for enhancing memory. Rosemary shouldn't be used during pregnancy or if you have high blood pressure. The safest rosemary essential oil is from Tunisia, North Africa.)

- Orange blossom

AROMATHERAPY IN YOUR KITCHEN

Judith Ben Hurley, herb specialist and author of *The Good Herb* and *Healing Secrets of the Seasons,* suggests that you add tea-making and juicing to your aromatherapy methods.

RELAXANTS

- Chamomile (Make chamomile tea and while drinking, breathe in the aroma.)

- Marjoram (Marjoram is an oregano-like herb. Put one teaspoon of dried marjoram in a cup of just-boiled water, cover and steep for four minutes, then sip slowly and breathe in the aroma.)

ENERGIZERS

- Orange (Squeeze a glass of fresh orange juice in the morning. While drinking your O.J., breathe in the reviving aroma.)

- Lemon (In the morning, squeeze the juice of half a lemon into a cup of hot water, sip slowly, and inhale the aroma. The drink may help you feel more energized.)

- Peppermint (For centuries Egyptians have depended on peppermint's stimulating aroma and recommended it to start the day. To begin your day with an herbal peppermint tea, try this ancient technique: at night, put one handful of fresh peppermint leaves in four cups of room-temperature water, cover, and let sit overnight. In the morning, discard the leaves and drink the refreshing water.)

Space

Ever wonder why some rooms invite you to work and others seem to suck energy from your body? Practitioners of the ancient Chinese art of feng shui will tell you it all has to do with invisible living energy, called "chi," and understanding the energy flow of a place. The ancient Chinese art of feng shui finds and creates balance and harmony in living and working environments. Ask yourself: Does the space you are in suck up your energy, or does it give you back energy? There's a tiny sushi shop around the block from the *Today* show. The customers' space isn't much more than eight by fourteen. It's far from elegant, but the space feels so good that it invites you back time and again. Says Sarah Shurety, who runs a feng shui company and recommends feng shui for Ten Downing Street, the English prime minister's residence: "The prime minister is the captain of the ship. His energy has got to be spot on. If he goes off course, the whole country goes off course." Robin Cook, the famous author who spends hours working out of his home office, told me that one reason for his success is having a well-constructed work space. He emphasizes this to such an extent that last time after speaking with him I noticed what a messy, uncomfortable work space I myself had grown accustomed to — on one side my wife's desk piled high with old newspapers, unpaid bills, moldering cups half drained of protein drink, on the other side my three-year-old's sofa littered with chewed toys, sticky candy wrappers, and broken crayons. I searched for help and found general feng shui principles that transformed my work space into a place of renewed productivity. These feng shui principles will allow you to design your own work space in the best possible way for your intended activity.

Although the principles of feng shui sound terrific, putting them into practice can be extraordinarily difficult. I read all I could, consulted with masters, read through the information on the Web, all without much success. However, in New Zealand I finally found the person I was looking for — Richard Webster, a feng shui expert and author of *Feng Shui for Beginners, 101 Feng Shui Tips for the Home,* and *Feng Shui in the Workplace.* His easy steps are the best I have found anywhere. Most of what follows are his recommendations for the location, shape, and layout of your office. Here are the dos and don'ts of creating a perfect work space.

Clutter

Don't clutter, because it will constrict "chi," or the flow of energy throughout the office. You should put away objects you're not using on a regular basis. Until you clear the clutter in your office, your whole life will feel cluttered. Boy, has this made a big difference in my life! I've been the king of clutter. Now I sweep away everything I'm not working on. Put a sofa or chairs in your office only if you're going to use them; otherwise they become clutter. If you have a bookshelf, fill it only with books you will actually be reading.

Electrical and computer cables

Keep electrical and computer cables out of sight, since the sight of electric cables will remind you of water (and water means wealth) being drained away.

Windows and lighting

- Have at least one window in your office, since windows allow "chi," or life force, into the room. Ideally, the windows should let sunlight in.

- Have good lighting. Light attracts "chi," so your whole office should be well lit. Good lighting will enhance your creativity and thinking. Put one light on or beside your desk to illuminate what you are doing, and place other lights around the room. Since dark corners create negative "chi," make sure your office does not have dark gloomy corners.

Wall decorations

- Use mirrors to make your office look larger.

- Hang paintings that you find personally appealing and hang them where you can see them, so they will positively affect your mood.

Colors

Choose colors that you find pleasing. Something black or blue (could be ornamental) is good, because in feng shui black and blue relate to the water element, which relates to money. Anything metallic or painted white activates the metallic element, which also relates to money. Something red activates the fire element, which relates to energy and excitement. Something green or wooden (e.g., plants or flowers) enhances the wood element, which relates to creativity and growth. Subtle and soothing color schemes are better than bright ones because bright ones could overly excite and negatively affect the moods of your visitors.

Plants

Choose live plants for your office. Don't choose dried plants with all water removed. Keep in mind that feng shui means "wind and water" ("feng" is the Chinese character for wind; "shui" means water).

The desk

- Don't sit with a window directly behind you at your desk, because when sitting at the desk, you will feel "lacking in support."

- Do get the biggest desk you can. Size is reflective of the status of the person sitting behind the desk. Have you noticed, for example, that in a company the president often has the largest desk? But beyond that, a large desk allows you the biggest expanse for your ideas and projects.

- If there are a number of people working in the office, don't face your desk toward another person, because that's confrontational. When possible, place the desks diagonal to one another, in a *pa-kua* shape (an octagon or eight-sided shape), which in feng shui is thought to create good energy because it covers all eight compass directions. You can also create a row of desks, so long as the sharp edges of the desks do not send "shars" or "poison arrows" to one another — you can counteract the creation of "shars" by using potted plants and dividers between desks.

- Do situate your desk so you can see anyone walking down the corridor or through the door. To maximize your overview, the desk should be as far away from the door as possible. The best place for your desk is usually diagonally across from the door — that gives you a commanding view of the room and the door, and in feng shui is called the Command Position or Power Position. Not only does the Power Position enable you to see, it also allows you to be seen, which is important so that you're not overlooked for promotions or pay rises. The desk should not be directly facing the door because that's intimidating to people coming into the office.

- Don't sit with your back to the door, since you will feel uncomfortable and vulnerable (in feng shui thought, you'd be exposed to being "stabbed in the back").

Location of your office

- Don't take an office at the end of a long corridor. Why? In feng shui a long corridor creates a "shar" or "poison arrow," which increases the potential of something bad happening.

- Don't take an office opposite a bathroom, because bathrooms create negative "chi" — since in feng shui water is wealth, a place that flushes away water creates negative "chi."

- Don't take an office facing a stairway going downward, because that symbolically means downward progress. It is fine, however, if your office faces a stairway going upward, because that can represent upward progress.

- Do take an office that is off the side of a corridor.

- Do take an office that is square or oblong

- Don't take an unusually shaped office — the angles can create a "shar."

Those are the basics. Now to follow to the limit the principles of feng shui in the office, divide your office into areas of wealth, fame, and career.

Area of wealth

When you enter the office, diagonally to the left as far back as you're able to walk is the wealth area. To activate the wealth area, place there something that relates to business and money. Since in feng shui the metallic element relates to money, anything metallic would activate the wealth area — you could use a small silver knickknack or something ornamental relating to money. (In Asia, people often hang on the walls of the wealth area coins interconnected with a red thread, the red being for good luck. Alternately, Asians often put in the wealth area an aquarium filled with eight goldfish and one black fish; such an aquarium strongly activates the wealth element, since the number eight relates to money, gold relates to money, and water also relates to money. The black fish is for protection against any disasters.)

Area of fame

The middle area of your office is the fame area. You should activate the fame area because it will increase your reputation and standing. In the fame area hang diplomas, certificates, or any photographs you have of yourself with someone accomplished in your field.

Area of career

When you come into your office, immediately to your right or left (depending on the location of the door) is the career area. Activate the career area by placing there something relating to your career, for example, a fax machine or a printer.

What a difference in productivity! My office now invites me in to work, to be creative. I don't have much space — my wife gave me the smallest room in our apartment. But cleared of clutter, and only a few hundred dollars later, I designed a space that boosts my mood and adds to my sense of wealth.

If you're a road warrior, take the time to create the perfect travel companions with just the right laptop, software, briefcases, and toilet kit. Take extra care to have nice pens and accessories that allow you to set up and feel at home wherever you are.

The bottom line is that your personal environment does matter. The difference between a good performance and a spectacular one is often minute. In the 100-meter dash, only a fraction of a second separates the performance of the world-record holder from that of an average athlete. Only a few carefully chosen words and gestures separate a middling salesman from a superior one. Small, seemingly insignificant changes can make all the difference in your performance, in your level of success, and in how you feel about yourself. Changing the space around you can produce a tremendous payoff for your general health and performance level. But remember, when you optimize conditions for a group, only 80 percent of people can be satisfied. You should be able to control as many factors as possible in your own environment in order to achieve an optimum work performance. The drive to put more people into fewer square feet is forcing people into more open offices, which is eliminating personal control. Since different people require different optimum conditions, shared office space is limiting. And the degree of control you have over your work environment will affect your health, mood, and productivity. Don't think you're acting like a grouse, or not being a team player, by speaking up about the space you work in. Change the space you work in; you'll be astounded at how good you'll feel.

So arrange your environment to boost your productivity and creativity. Pay attention to temperature, air quality, light, sound, smell, and space. Create an atmosphere that is feng shui positive, that brings you luck and good fortune. Design a space that you love and a space that will love you back; and experience the magic and miracle of place.

Step 3: Turn On the Tunes

||||||

Last summer my wife and I were enjoying the magic of the Côte d'Azur. A mistral wind from the Sahara had blown every last trace of dust and humidity from the atmosphere. It appeared you could see forever. Then came the call from our network Foreign Desk. America had bombed Sudan, a country I had reported on for over a decade. I was asked to fly immediately to Africa to cover the event. I packed my bags, leaving one of the most treasured places on earth for the middle of the Sahara, Khartoum, according to American officials the heart of the Islamic terrorist empire. My wife was in tears, our vacation in tatters. I was up at 4:30 the next morning for a quick bike ride, then packed for an 8 A.M. flight to Nice and on to Zurich, Cairo, and Khartoum. With four hours of sleep and thoughts drifting to my young children at home in Vermont and my poor wife packing to leave, my mood was somewhere below sewer level. But after a quick nap on the airplane, I plugged my earphones into the airplane sound system. Out poured *The Marriage of Figaro,* the stunning Mozart opera . . . in minutes my mood was soaring. The change was no accident.

Music has remarkable properties that can propel you toward success. Think of how your imagination soared when you were cruising the local strip as a teenager with the radio blasting the latest top ten hits. Anything seemed possible. The sky was the limit. Remember how much faster your heart raced during runs or aerobics classes when music was added. Recall the grand and noble thoughts that seemed to flow while you were listening to a great symphony. Music's effect isn't just happenstance. Researchers appreciate the tremendous motivational power of music, with its ability to lift your spirits and even improve your intelligence. The therapeutic use of music is a well-developed and extremely effective means of controlling your mental energy throughout the day: when you first jump out of bed, on the drive to work, when exercising or in the office.

>**CONVENTIONAL WISDOM:** Music is entertain-
>ment.
>**THE BIOLOGY OF SUCCESS:** Music is genius.

The strategic choice of the right music will pull you kicking and dragging from a foul mood to a good one; using music, you can alter, monitor, and "customize" your mood to help you achieve the task at hand. This chapter will help you carefully select what to play and when.

Music and the Biology of Success

Music effects positive changes in our psychological, physical, cognitive, and social functions. Because music accesses so many different parts of the brain, its effect is profound on our emotional and physical lives and therefore on our quest for success. In the brain, music is processed in the amygdala, a part of the so-called limbic system that is closely associated with emotions and imagery — and so music directly stimulates our emotions and imagery. Music also has a direct effect on the body; rhythm, for example, is processed in the same parts of the brain that control heart rate and blood pressure. Music is as efficient and quick as other established methods of relaxation such as meditation or yoga. Music can bust high stress levels as well as induce muscle relaxation. In fact, music reduces stress so effectively that stress hormone levels actually sink. In his book *Messengers of Paradise: Opiates and the Brain,* Charles Levinthal explains how the process of listening can release endorphins that can alleviate pain and induce euphoria. Music can even potentially boost your immune system. Cheryl Dileo, Ph.D., Professor of Music Therapy, and her colleagues at Temple University in Philadelphia, Pennsylvania, looked at a disease-fighting antibody, called IgA, found in saliva. "We found that in participants, twenty minutes of listening to music significantly increased their IgA levels." These aren't just random observations; music is a force so powerful that doctors use it in treatment.

Already in the sixteenth century, in *Gargantua and Pantagruel,* the French poet Rabelais described the success obtained with music therapy; Rabelais wrote of a queen who could "'cure any and all illnesses without touching anyone, simply by playing the sick an appropriate song.'"* In 1571, spa patients took singing therapy at the German resort of Aachen. By 1773, the hospital Ospedale Santo Spirito in Rome played organ music for its patients. But the World Wars gave music therapy its biggest boost, when both amateur and professional musicians played for the thousands of veterans suffering both the physical and the emotional trauma of war. The patients showed remarkable physical and emotional improvements in response to the music, and so hospitals started to hire musicians on a regular basis. However, it was soon evident that hospital musicians needed some prior training before entering the medical facility, and so demand for a college curriculum grew. The first music therapy degree program in the world was founded at Michigan State University in 1944. The National Association for Music Therapy was founded in 1950.

Music is so effective as therapy that hospitals throughout Western Europe and the United States use music therapy to sedate or induce sleep, to counteract apprehension or fear, to lessen muscle tension for the purpose of relaxation, and, in conjunction with anesthesia or pain medication, to alleviate pain. Many top surgeons play music in the operating room for the benefit of both doctors and patients. Music therapy is an effective psychotherapeutic treatment to elevate depressed patients' moods and help the severely mentally ill, for example patients suffering from schizophrenia, borderline disorders, or severe mental handicaps.

Music therapists design customized music sessions based on an individual's emotional well-being, physical health, social func-

---

*François Rabelais, *Gargantua and Pantagruel,* trans. Burton Raffel (New York: W. W. Norton, 1990), p. 564.

tioning, communication abilities, and cognitive skills, all assessed through actual responses to different kinds of music. Then they prescribe music improvisation, receptive music listening, song writing, lyric discussion, music and imagery, music performance, and learning through music.

How to Elevate Your Mood with Music Therapy

To put this theory to work, find music that matches your current mood, regardless of what it is: depressed, neutral, sad, or angry. Then, using three or four different songs or melodies, gradually change the kind of music over a twenty-minute period to the way you want to feel. You will find that your mood will change with the change in music. Ideally, you'll make a tape with the songs in the order that works best for you or program a CD to play the songs in the correct order. Says Dr. Dileo, "That's an important strategy. If we can match the stimulus and then change it, the mood changes." How to choose the music? "Experts take into account the melody, rhythm, harmony, and timbre, but amateurs can just look at how it makes them feel. Music will change you. Even if you like sad music because it's letting you indulge in your bad feelings, force yourself to change the music to upbeat, happy music and your mood will be uplifted. Music is very complex but the way it works is very simple. The key is to end with a piece of music that you want to reflect your desired mood."

This technique to alter mood is based on the iso-moodic principle, a theory that dates back to the Greeks. Iso-moodic means "same mood" and refers to the principle of beginning treatment by matching the music to your existing mood and ending with music that reflects your desired mood at the end of the session. When should you employ this iso-moodic technique to change mood? Whenever you want. Dr. Dileo says it has more to do with intent than anything else: "I think it should be done on an as-needed basis." If you have trouble getting out of bed, use it then. One wonderful aspect of music is that it's so very accessible. Headphones allow you full-time access. Afraid of an interview? Intimidated by a meeting with your boss? There's a good body of research that shows that music can help cut anxiety. Dr. Dileo says, "It's the iso-moodic principle again. Find music that matches how you are feeling and then change it over to relaxing music. If there's no time, just listen to the relaxing music. Focus all your attention on the music; it will take you away from anxiety-producing thoughts." For some people suffering from anxiety, music can help them to express their innermost needs.

Music is the most phenomenal library of human feelings; it's an amazing catalogue. Find what feels good — maybe for you it's the end of Stravinsky's *Rite of Spring*. When you find a piece that moves you, indulge in it. A good listener has a large library of musical devices in his head, but not all are developed. If you don't have the necessary structure for understanding in your brain, give the structures time and space to evolve by listening to a piece you like over and over again. And then go hunting for other examples. That's the best way — discover it for yourself so that you will keep doing it; just as a diet will not last without your loving the new eating habits, you're not going to keep listening if you don't love the music. But you need to push. What you hear is not all that's there; trust that there is more, and keep listening. The pleasure the music will eventually yield is unbelievable. You just need to explore until you find something that speaks to whatever part of your personality needs expression.

How do you select the right music? Professor Ellen Rosand, Ph.D., Chairwoman of the Music Department at Yale University, says that musicians throughout history have speculated about the mood effects of certain pieces. Ramon Satyendra, Ph.D., Associate Professor of Music at Yale University, and editor of the *Journal of Music Theory*, stresses that listening to music is a rich and varied experience that can go well beyond merely associating a specific mood with a given piece. He also says, however, that some special works were written to evoke or represent specific moods; he compiled for us the following list. You may want to try the pieces below and add them to your own favorites.

Lament: These pieces include a specific kind of descending bass line that connotes intense expression of mourning, grief, and tragedy.

- Henry Purcell: Dido's lament in *Dido and Aeneas* has a step-by-step descending chromatic bass line that became a prototype for subsequent composers depicting grief.

- Johann Sebastian Bach: Capriccio in B-flat

- Wolfgang Amadeus Mozart: Quartet in D-minor (K.421)

- Ludwig von Beethoven: 32 Variations in C-minor

Pastoral: These works contain passages that evoke the atmosphere of nature and rural life.

- Antonio Vivaldi: *The Four Seasons*

- Franz Joseph Haydn: *The Creation*

- Ludwig von Beethoven: Pastoral Symphony (Symphony No. 6) and the Pastoral Sonata for Piano (Sonata in D-major)

- Carl Maria von Weber: *Der Freischütz* (overture)

- Claude Debussy: Prelude to the Afternoon of a Faun

Madness: Sometimes composers have sought to represent extreme mental states such as bacchanalian frenzy or agitated confusion.

- Hector Berlioz: *Symphonie fantastique*

- Arnold Schoenberg: *Pierrot Lunaire*

Apotheosis: In these works, a dramatic effect, usually near the end, gives a sense of apotheosis. A striking moment of resolution coinciding with a sudden change of musical character signals the moment of apotheosis — maybe the theme returns or all instruments sound at the same time, or a key comes back.

- Wolfgang Amadeus Mozart: The finale in the Jupiter Symphony (Symphony No. 41)

- Franz Liszt: The "Chorus Mysticus" in the Faust Symphony

- Ludwig von Beethoven: The "Ode to Joy" in Symphony No. 9
- Richard Wagner: The death of Brunhilde at the end of *Götterdämmerung*

Finally, below is a selection of music compositions you can rely on to change your mood, perhaps elevate it or even bring it to a crescendo and keep it there. Explore the list at your leisure; pick those pieces that work for you and discard those that fail.

Johann Sebastian Bach
- Two-Part Inventions
- The Well-Tempered Clavier
- "The French Suites"
- "The English Suites"
- The Art of the Fugue

George Frederick Handel
- Oratorios
- *Messiah*
- Ceremonial Music for Trumpet and Organ

Wolfgang Amadeus Mozart
- Symphonies
- Five violin concertos
- *The Magic Flute*
- *The Marriage of Figaro*
- *La Clemenza di Tito*

Franz Joseph Haydn
- String quartets

Ludwig von Beethoven
- Symphonies Nos. 1–9
- Late string quartets
- Piano sonatas
- Violin concertos
- Piano Concerto, "The Emperor"

Johannes Brahms
- Symphonies Nos. 1–4
- Intermezzos for Solo Piano
- Hungarian Dances

Franz Schubert
- Songs

Robert Schumann
- Piano music
- Songs

Frédéric Chopin
- Preludes
- Nocturnes

Antonín Dvořák
- Symphony No. 9, "From the New World"
- Slavonic Dances

Claude Debussy
- *La Mer*
- G-Minor String Quartet

Igor Stravinsky
- *Petrushka*
- *Firebird*

Béla Bartók
- Concerto for Orchestra
- String quartets

Boosting Cognition

In an experiment published in 1993, Frances H. Rauscher, Assistant Professor of Cognitive Development, and her colleagues at the University of California, Irvine, reported that listening to Mozart (compared to silence or just following relaxation instructions) produced in college students a brief but significant increase in performance of a spatial IQ task involving mental manipulations of folded cut paper.* After some criticism, Dr. Rauscher replicated and extended her findings.** In this newer study, she used the same task as in her first experiment but extended the types of listening experienced. Seventy-nine college students were divided into three groups, each of which listened to one of the following: silence, Mozart's Sonata for Two Pianos, K.448 (the same piece that produced the positive results in the 1993 study), and a minimalist work by Philip Glass. Only the Mozart group showed a significant increased spatial IQ score. Dr. Rauscher also found that listening to a taped short story or dance music did not enhance test scores. Therefore, improving a measure of spatial IQ seemed to be specific to some aspect of Mozart's music, or of other complex music with similar features.

Some are skeptical of what has become known as the "Mozart Effect." Professor Satyendra, who is interested in the neurobiology of the musical experience, cautions us not to overinterpret the results of the study in which people who listened to Mozart performed better on intelligence tests: "It's tempting to conclude that listening to a genius turns us into geniuses; this interpretation plays into a fascination with the 'genius figure,' which has been part of European and American culture since the nineteenth century." But he does emphasize that music enhances intelligence in all sorts of

---

*F. H. Rauscher, G. L. Shaw, and K. N. Ky, "Music and Spatial Task Performance," *Nature* 365 (1993): 611.
**F. H. Rauscher, G. L. Shaw, and K. N. Ky, "Listening to Mozart Enhances Spatial-Temporal Reasoning: Towards a Neurophysiological Basis," *Neuroscience Letters* 185 (1995): 44–47.

ways: "A young child sight-reading violin music is being challenged simultaneously at the tactile, visual, auditory, and intellectual levels. Music is unique in the extent to which it engages and disciplines a child's cognitive skills."

Why Classical Music

So, why classical music? I like rock and pop as much as everyone else and use those genres often to boost my mood. The trouble is it's just plain hard to get a real, sustained high with rock/pop. You may feel really pumped while playing pop or rock, but there is a quick let-down as you look for more. A great deejay might keep you going for twenty minutes, but then it ends. That makes rock 'n' roll the crack of music enjoyment. Robert Jourdain, composer and author of *Music, the Brain, and Ecstasy,* explains why: "You experience much larger structures in classical music. Just as comic books are not as good as Shakespeare, the Rolling Stones are not nearly as good as Bach or Mozart or Beethoven. Why do we care about comprehending larger things, understanding complexity? Well, because that's the essence of the intelligence that makes us human." Only music that is well developed at a certain level will have a large, complex structure. Music gives us a structure of understanding by creating relations across time, and that structure, if successfully modeled, gives pleasure.

How does music yield pleasure? We can experience the deepest pleasures of classical music only when our minds have learned to anticipate and perceive such large structures. The key principle is the "implication-realization" model, which creates an anticipation and then satisfies by fulfilling that anticipation. A memorable example is the famous choral conclusion of Beethoven's Ninth. Leonard B. Meyer and Eugene Narmour, professors of music at the University of Pennsylvania, developed the "implication-realization" model of musical process, a theory that addresses listeners' expectations of resolution. It's a psychological theory of music that considers how music is built in terms of implication and realization, tension and resolution. In *Music, the Brain, and Ecstasy,* Jourdain compares this satisfaction to lovemaking: "Well-written music takes its good time satisfying anticipations. It teases, repeatedly instigating an anticipation and hinting at its satisfaction . . . only to hold back with a false cadence. . . . If this process sounds as much like the recipe for good lovemaking as for good music-making, it's because the nervous system functions the same way in all its reaches."* Jourdain says he uses the term "ecstasy" because "ecstasy arises as a brain models large structures, as it discovers deep relations in the world. Ecstasy emerges when you reach a higher level of comprehension. You get a second jolt when you find that you have transcended yourself — you become smarter, have a larger moment of awareness. When we enter that state, we are amazed. What makes art different from ordinary experience is that it creates an artificial environment that can push the brain to levels of comprehension far beyond what we find in everyday life."

So, which classical music works best? Mozart is more popular than other classical composers because he has strong, charming melodies that can hold the listener captive; but you should not listen exclusively to Mozart. In this chapter I suggest a number of classical composers, and, as your repertoire expands, you'll find pleasure in all. Expert music therapists will tell you that no one particular style of music is more therapeutic than another, and that typical music therapy sessions are designed and music selected based on the individual client's treatment plan. In choosing musical selections for you, however, I have concentrated on classical pieces, partly because of the results gleaned from the Mozart experiments, and partly because of the general consensus that classical music is relationally much deeper than rock and pop, which is mostly surface effects and volume.

---

*Robert Jourdain, *Music, the Brain, and Ecstasy* (New York: Avon Books, 1998), p. 319.

Learning to Appreciate Classical Music

Appreciating a variety of musical styles calls on the listener to develop different listening strategies. Becoming skilled at recognizing different types of patterns and organization allows you better to savor what different musical styles have to offer. Just as you naturally recognize words and idioms without focusing on individual letters, in the act of listening you can naturally discern composite units, such as whole melodies and phrases. The more kinds of organization and patterning you can appreciate, the more receptive you will be to different kinds of music. Professor Satyendra suggests to the interested listener the following list for practice in hearing certain musical elements:

Simultaneous melodies

- Johann Sebastian Bach: *The Art of the Fugue* and *The Well-Tempered Clavier*

- Johannes Brahms: A German Requiem and the Fourth Symphony

Formal architecture (the effective balancing of large sections of music against one another in order to create a pleasing whole)

- Ludwig von Beethoven: Third Symphony and "Hammerklavier" Sonata for Piano

- Anton Bruckner: Seventh and Ninth symphonies

- Franz Schubert: String Quintet in C-Major, and the "Great" C-Major Symphony

Rich, complex chord progressions

- César Franck: D-Minor Symphony and the chorales for organ

- Sergey Rachmaninoff: *The Isle of the Dead,* symphonic poem for orchestra, and the *Etudes-tableaux* for piano

- Frédéric Chopin: Ballades for piano

Blending of the sounds of orchestral instruments

- Richard Strauss: Tone poems for orchestra

- Gustav Mahler: Third and Eighth symphonies

- Maurice Ravel: *Daphnis et Chloé*

Music that pushes the limits of the common-practice tonality classical period

- Claude Debussy: Preludes for piano

- Arnold Schoenberg: *Gurrelieder* and the First Chamber Symphony

- Béla Bartók: Concerto for Orchestra, and the Divertimento for Strings

Exotic scales and the unusual harmonies that can be derived from them

- Igor Stravinsky: *Firebird* and *The Rite of Spring*

- Alexander Scriabin: Piano music

If you don't currently listen to much classical music, try classical-music-compilation CDs known as "greatest hits" CDs. You'll get a good mix of piano, string quartets, and orchestral music. At first try to find collections including as many of the composers listed above as possible. If you want an overview of Mozart's music, you might consider Dan Campbell's compilation CD *The Mozart Effect*.

To improve your listening skills you can do more than just listen to music. Improving your listening skills is called ear training. Experts agree that singing is one of the most important components of ear training. Singing is the most direct musical expression — take singing lessons, join a choir, sing with a friend. You can also develop your listening by learning an instrument: take piano lessons, learn to improvise on the keyboard, learn an instrument that corresponds to what you want to learn to listen to. We bought a piano for ourselves and our children. You don't have to become an accomplished player; even at a novice level, you'll be training your ear.

Synergy

You can boost the effect of music therapy by exercising or deep breathing to music or actually singing along.

Exercise

You'll find that you will work out harder longer when you use the correct tempo music to exercise. Since exercise is already lifting your mood, the additional input of music produces a terrific synergy. Energizing music is a big reason that spin and aerobics classes are so popular.

Deep breathing

"If you're experiencing anxiety, follow the rhythm of the music when you breathe," says Dr. Dileo. "We see changes even when we ask people just to observe their breathing without trying to change it. This enhances a meditative state."

Singing

"Singing addresses the mind and body simultaneously," says Dr. Dileo. Singing embodies the perfect marriage of improved mood and cognition with decreased anxiety. Singing along with great music delivers a great feel-good mood. I've memorized Zarastro's passages from Mozart's *Magic Flute* in order to sing in the shower or along with the CD.

Go ahead. Do it! Buy that sound system you always wanted. I keep some kind of music-playing device close at hand: a radio in my bedroom, a CD player for exercising, another CD player in the car, and a third in the office. Always travel with a Discman or tape player. Set up your office, home, and bedroom with a sound system. The new 200 CD jukebox changers are a terrific way to store the tunes that get you going. So go ahead — take the time and turn on the tunes!

Step 4: Eat for Mental Energy

I used to feel miserable after a week on the road — tense, anxious, tired, and generally unproductive. After years of research into high-performance nutrition, I now feel terrific, even on a heavy travel schedule, the best I've ever felt. In October–November 1998, I was in twenty-five cities and half a dozen countries in just twenty-eight days. Not only did I feel great, I actually lost weight. By understanding the principles of high-performance nutrition, you can add hours of high-level productivity to your day and still keep your waistline trim.

> **CONVENTIONAL WISDOM:** Pack in the carbs to perform.
> **THE BIOLOGY OF SUCCESS:** Create success one meal at a time through the foods you eat.

The Biology of Nutrition

Great nutrition is one of the few measures that increase both the production of key neurotransmitters responsible for mood and your level of alertness.

For generations, we've believed that altering levels of brain chemicals required psychoactive drugs or psychotropic medications. The great breakthrough came when researchers found that by supplying the building blocks of these brain chemicals through the foods we eat, we could build higher stores of specific brain chemicals that, in turn, change our mood. This work was largely carried out by pioneers Dr. Judith Wurtman of McLean Hospital, one of Harvard Medical School's teaching hospitals, and Dr. Richard Wurtman of the Massachusetts Institute of Technology.

There are two key neurotransmitters you can affect with food. First, you can improve alertness by eating protein. As proteins are digested, an amino acid called tyrosine is absorbed by the bloodstream and delivered to the brain. Tyrosine is a key building block for alertness neurotransmitters, the most powerful of which is dopamine. Tyrosine is powerful enough that it's been recommended to the armed forces by the National Academy of Sciences and has been used by bomber pilots to help them remain alert and awake for long bombing runs. However, tyrosine has to compete with other amino acids to gain entrance to the brain. Tyrosine's most notable competitor is another amino acid, tryptophan, found in carbohydrates. If protein is eaten alone or with a very limited quantity of carbohydrate, tyrosine gains ready access to the brain. Too many carbohydrates, and tryptophan wins the competition, drowning out the effect of protein by restricting the entrance of tyrosine into the brain.

Second, you can induce a calming effect by eating foods very high in carbohydrate. As carbohydrates are digested, tryptophan is absorbed by the bloodstream and delivered to the brain. Tryptophan is a key building block of the neurotransmitter serotonin. Serotonin is a powerful antidepressant and has a strong calming effect. However, too much serotonin goes beyond calming to downright sleep inducing!

Tactics

Timing your intake of foods for mental performance is critical. Foods are powerful medicines. Most of us take them blindly and suffer the consequences. In my book *Dr. Bob Arnot's Revolutionary Weight Control Program,* I advocated "Feedforward Eating," an effective concept that relies on your intellect and judgment to time eating the right foods for the right performance.

Feedforward Eating means consuming the right foods in advance of a meeting, a workout, a nap, or a concentrated intellectual effort so that you feel and perform exactly as you want. With Feedforward Eating, you plan your day according to how you want to feel at a given time or for a specific activity. You then eat foods that will make you feel the way you want when you want. Feedforward Eating takes the immense arsenal of foods that act as drugs and projects it powerfully forward in time. By understanding in advance exactly how you would like to feel and perform, you can extract the maximum help from foods. In this way you can redirect your body's physiology toward that of weight loss, kill your hunger before you become hungry, and make your brain feel great so that depression, anxiety, restlessness, craving, or bingeing don't ruin your day and your diet. If you're trying to loose weight, the feeling to go for is lean but not hungry.

Carbohydrates

Be wary of carbo overload. Too many of the wrong carbos dull mental performance and alertness.

Carbohydrates have very different effects on performance at different times of day and different times of the month.

- Carbohydrate in the morning can quickly bring your blood sugar up from its overnight low. That's critical if you're going to exercise first thing in the morning. However, too big a dose of carbohydrates for breakfast, especially when you are not exercising, starts the day with mental dullness.

- Excess carbos at lunch can also make you sleepy and groggy.

- Carbos in the late afternoon, however, can cut and soothe the tension that rises to its height at 4:00–5:00 P.M. and restore calm when alertness is at a low anyhow. That's why at 4:00 P.M. in our *Dateline* offices, producers and correspondents make a beeline for the little bowls of candy strategically placed around the office.

- At night, a modest amount of the right carbos can help you fall asleep.

What are the right carbos? Carbohydrates that don't cause a large increase in blood sugar levels — in other words, carbos with a low glycemic index. High-glycemic or fast-release carbohydrates break down quickly and quickly give rise to high blood sugars that place a heavy glucose load on your body. These do build more serotonin more quickly, but at a price. You may quickly experience a "sugar high"; but the surges in blood sugar that these carbos deliver can be followed by a sense of feeling jittery and even depressed as blood sugar crashes. I try to avoid starches and refined grains as a way of limiting carbo overload and controlling my weight. Beans, vegetables, many fruits, and high-fiber foods are the carbohydrates you can eat that have the least effect on blood sugar. To help you choose the right carbos, I've included in the workbook on pages 215–218 tables of high-, moderate-, and low-glucose carbos. Keep in mind we often eat for emotional reasons, and the foods we are most likely to abuse are those that hit pleasure centers in the brain, for example fast-release carbos. Eating for emotional reasons goes something like this: "I've had a bad day — I want a pint of ice cream," or "I have to study all night; I want chocolate to cheer me up and help me focus," when in reality a tuna salad with spinach would make you more alert and help you study better!

Although I've just cautioned against fast-release carbodydrates, there are two highly specialized tactical uses of fast-release carbohydrates. The first is as a treatment for PMS. Sugary foods or drinks do relieve some of the psychic distress of PMS. However, drugs such as Prozac, taken just during those critical days of each month, may be a lower-calorie approach. Second, ingested immediately before or during intense aerobic exercise, a beverage containing fast-release carbohydrates may improve performance. Adding 15 percent protein powder to these high-performance drinks can keep you from feeling sleepy or losing concentration during exercise. This is especially valuable just before a morning workout.

Protein

Besides energizing the brain, protein also satiates more quickly and effectively than either carbohydrate or fat. With such traits, it is no wonder that protein has become the most commercially successful food group for dieters.

You can use protein strategically to maximize your mental and physical energy throughout the day. Here's how:

- Eat some protein at the beginning of each meal to satiate your hunger in order to prevent overeating.

- Use higher protein concentrations in the morning and for lunch to make your workday more productive.

- Use a protein supplement in your sports drink to increase endurance and concentration.

- Use protein in the evening only if you have to be sharp and alert.

So spread your protein intake throughout the day according to how you need to feel at different times of the day. Of course your protein need will vary depending on your weight and level of activity. The workbook contains a table (pages 218–219) to help you determine your level of physical activity and the number of grams of protein that you should be ingesting.

Also in the workbook is a list of the leanest proteins (pages 219–224).

Fats

FATS TO EAT: OMEGA-3S

Researchers have good reason to call fish "brain food." The most important fats in fish are called omega-3 fatty acids. Found in cold-saltwater fish, the omega-3 fatty acids, nicknamed omega-3s, serve the fish as an insulator against cold water. For humans, whose brains are roughly 60 percent fat, omega-3s are widely heralded as a means of promoting optimum brain performance. Michael A. Schmidt, Ph.D., author of *Smart Fats* and Visiting Professor of Applied Biochemistry and Clinical Nutrition at Northwestern College, says: "Eating specific essential fatty acids transforms who we are by affecting the brain's vital functions. The brain cannot make essential fatty acids, which must come from our diet. Humans evolved on diets containing substantially more omega-3 essential fatty acids than we consume in typical Western diets. The kinds and amounts of fatty acids consumed may be important in numerous psychiatric and neurological disorders ranging from learning and behavioral disorders in children to both major and bipolar depression as well as schizophrenia in adults. Preliminary studies indicate that an imbalance of essential fatty acid intake may well relate to such problems as social violence, aggressive behavior, and suicide."

In September 1998, the National Institutes of Health (NIH) sponsored a workshop on omega-3 essential fatty acids in psychiatric disorders in order to stimulate hard-nosed clinical testing in this new and developing field. Investigators presented data showing that consuming omega-3 fatty acids reduced troublesome symptoms in schizophrenia and manic-depressive disorders. Joseph R. Hibbeln, M.D., of the National Institute on Alcohol Abuse and Alcoholism, one of the National Institutes of Health, confirmed that omega-3s may well have a role in the treatment of major depression by regulating levels of brain serotonin. He noted that countries in which people consume higher amounts of fish, a source of omega-3s, have lower rates of major depression and postpartum depression. Dr. Andrew Stoll of McLean Hospital and Harvard Medical School found that taking fish oil supplements could markedly reduce symptoms of manic-depressive illness. He found that twelve of fourteen patients remained free of depression or mania when omega-3 fatty acids were added to their diet, compared to only six of sixteen patients who received only a dummy pill. These doctors caution, however, that patients should remain on their current medication and consult their physician before taking these fatty acids.

How do omega-3 fatty acids affect serotonin function? Two omega-3 fatty acids, EPA (eicosapentaenoic acid) and DHA (docosahexaenoic acid), may change serotonin function in a way that decreases violent, depressive, and even suicidal behavior. Just as we've learned that tyrosine and tryptophan can increase dopamine and serotonin production, ingesting omega-3 fats affects the signals between nerves by changing the "brain's synaptic membranes." Here's what that means. Neurotransmitters are released from the end of one nerve, travel across a narrow space, and then signal another nerve. Fatty acids are the principal structural molecules that make up the nerve ending; and the membranes at all synapses are particularly rich in the long-chain fatty acids — especially arachidonic acid and an omega-3 fat called DHA. There is evidence that the integrity of the fatty acids at the synapse affects the shape of the receptors; if there are not enough fatty acids or the wrong kind of fatty acids, the receptor's shape can change, and with the changed shape it becomes harder for the neurotransmitters, such as dopamine, to bind. Restoring the fatty acid balance will restore the shape. There is some evidence that the fatty acid levels and ratios affect the neurotransmitter levels themselves. Fatty acids may also affect mood through the eicosanoids. The observation that rates of depression are lower in countries where more fish is consumed is consistent with these changes in neurotransmitter function.

Without the completion of further clinical trials, you may wonder where this leaves us. The important key is that Western diets have sharply less fish oils than they did in the last century. During this same time depression has increased nearly a hundredfold. That link is still not enough to recommend fish oils for pure mental performance purposes. However, researchers think that fish oils are the heart-healthiest fat and may play a strong preventive role against breast cancer. Both the British and Canadian governments have recommended daily minimum intakes of fish oils. For that reason I advocate fish oils, primarily for general health reasons and secondarily for their effect on the brain. Make sure you regularly include fish in your diet. If you want to take fish oil capsules, first consult with your doctor.

A table in the workbook (pages 224–225) shows the total amount of omega-3 fatty acids in various fish and fish oils. Look for the omega-3 fatty acids EPA and DHA. They are the most critically important omega-3 fatty acids found in fish. The table lists the amount of EPA and DHA plus their total.

Supplements

There are dozens of supplements touted for improved mental performance. I don't find enough data to recommend wholeheartedly any of them. Caffeine does cause a short-term improvement in mental performance, and small amounts in the morning might be useful, especially if you have slept poorly. The most interesting new evidence is for ginkgo biloba. Published data suggests that extracts of ginkgo biloba may improve the memory of Alzheimer's disease patients. Dr. Jeffrey Kaye of the Oregon Health Sciences University in Portland reported that patients who took 120 to 240 milligrams of ginkgo biloba for three to six months had a 3 percent increase in tests of memory and learning compared with those taking a placebo. The report, in the November 1998 issue of the *Archives of Neurology,* pooled the data from four studies with 424 patients. Some experts speculate that middle-aged men and women might acquire some protective benefit by taking ginkgo before memory problems develop. There is, however, no proof that this is true. If you take the blood-thinning medicine Coumadin, or aspirin, or have a bleeding disorder, be wary of taking ginkgo without your physician's approval.

Do's and Don'ts

Breakfast

Ever wonder how the English managed to build an empire on which the sun never set? I'd like to think it was a big hearty breakfast. Maybe part of England's decline is that so many Englishmen now eat the same skimpy continental breakfast as the Europeans!

DO:

• Have a high-protein start as soon as you're out of bed and at least twenty minutes before you eat the rest of your breakfast. Yogurt, fish, low-fat or skim milk, soy milk, soy protein powder or other protein powders mixed as healthy "smoothies" all provide good doses of protein. Of these, the most powerful are soy protein mixes because they have the greatest amount of tyrosine and can build the most alerting neurotransmitters fastest. Eggs also have a high-protein content. Have one or two yolks with four to six egg whites to get the most protein with the least added cholesterol. The egg whites will fill you up but are low in fat. A single egg for breakfast is not associated with an increased risk of heart disease or stroke, according to a recent Harvard study.

- After showering and dressing, eat your main breakfast. This should be a real "stick to your ribs" meal that will maintain low blood sugar levels and supply lots of energy while keeping you satiated. One and a half cups of high-fiber cereal, such as raw steel cut oatmeal, with yogurt or low-fat or skim milk, and a high-fiber fruit such as cantaloupe provide a great meal.

- Instead of coffee, try noncaffeinated teas as an energizing morning drink. The French recommend thyme tea, which is noncaffeinated; the Chinese recommend ginseng (not to be taken by pregnant women or people with high blood pressure). Black teas will give you some caffeine if you need it. The black tea Earl Grey contains essence of bergamot, which is an antidepressant.

DON'T:

- Eat high-fat foods such as bacon, sausages, or hash browns. Such foods dilute and delay the effect that great foods have on your brain chemistry.

- Eat foods that cause a large rise and fall in your blood sugar, such as donuts, danish, bagels, and white toast.

- Drink a lot of caffeine. If you crave it, hold off for a couple of hours after breakfast to see if you really need it. Your natural rise in alertness will come just from getting up and will be aided by a great breakfast. Avoid at all costs combining caffeine and quickly digested carbohydrates, like a coffee and white toast. Both sugar and caffeine provide a temporary fix, but the following spikes and troughs in insulin and glucose and the unavoidable crash will make you feel far worse than you did before you ate and drank. If caffeine and sugar are used throughout the day, over time they may create chronic fatigue, anxiety, and a low mood.

- Skip breakfast: Not eating at all robs your body of any chance to boost alertness or make the neurotransmitters that make you feel good and energetic. From a dieting viewpoint, you also save nothing. If you want to overeat, overeat at breakfast. With the right slow-release carbos and proteins, you'll increase the rate of calorie burn.

Morning snacks

DO:

- Eat fruit. This is a great time to have your fruit if you've missed it at breakfast, say half a cantaloupe, which gives you lots of fiber and antioxidants.

DON'T:

- Eat a pure carbohydrate snack. The big mistake most of us make is having a pure carbohydrate snack, which can lead to drowsiness and a low blood sugar. Bagels, donuts, cinnamon rolls, and toast for midmorning snacks just don't work.

Lunch

DO:

- Concentrate on a high-protein lunch. The decrease in mental alertness during the afternoon is a gradual slope, not a big dropoff. To keep the slope more gradual, eat high amounts of protein. Go for a large protein meal without going overboard on fat. What I like best is a big piece of lean fish because of the high-protein, low-fat content, and the beneficial properties of omega-3. Tuna (no mayo), turkey, or chicken are quick on-the-go alternatives.

- Try green leafy vegetables and legumes containing a high concentration of folate, which may have the added benefit of slowing the mental decline of aging.

- If you usually get hungry in the afternoon, add to your lunch a serving of beans for satiety and to stabilize your blood sugar.

- If you're a vegetarian, then a grain-bean combination gives you 95 percent of all your micro- and macronutrients. By having more beans, especially tyrosine-rich soybeans, and fewer grains, you'll reap more from the energizing effect of the protein. I'll have a serving of beans for lunch, with fresh vegetables on the side and a small amount of wild rice. This is a great way of eating some carbohydrates without creating mental dullness. Those carbos can slightly increase your metabolism to give you extra energy for physical activities during the afternoon.

- Drink lots of water to improve satiety.

DON'T:

- If you want to remain alert, don't eat starchy foods, such as pasta, potatoes, or breads, or sugary foods, all of which have a quick serotonin release that will cause mental fatigue. The mental dullness that follows may spur you to eat more and drink more caffeine, neither of which is necessary if you avoid starches.

Afternoon snacks

- If you've been craving carbs, now is the time to cash in, when you feel edgy and have lost your concentration in the mid to late afternoon. Try microwaving a small sweet potato at the same time every day in the late afternoon. The sweet potato is superhealthful and releases some serotonin, which combats the carbs craving. A black bean soup is an even better bet, because it releases sugar so slowly. If you do choose slow-release carbs, be sure to eat far enough in advance of your projected afternoon cravings to satisfy them. That will prevent you from lunging for a coworker's potato chips. Some cereals qualify as healthy snacks so long as they are high in fiber. Each food you put in your mouth should hit a few birds with one stone: controlling blood sugar, promoting the proper brain chemistry, and satisfying your hunger.

    The idea of late-in-the-day carbos was pioneered by Dr. Judith Wurtman, director of the TRIAD weight management center at McLean Hospital. Dr. Wurtman's basic plan is to give enough carbohydrate to increases brain serotonin levels and keep them high between 4:00 P.M. and bedtime, when many people feel most stressed. Her clients drink a carbohydrate beverage, which decreases stress and the tendency to eat more food in response to stress.

Dinner

DO:

- Eat a higher amount of carbohydrate. Concentrate on balance but with a higher concentration of carbohydrates to produce more serotonin and calm you for sleep. Dr. Judith Wurtman, who advocates having more carbohydrates at dinner, says that for maximum effectiveness you should have very little protein with the carbohydrates.

- Beware, though: Starches may kill your evening productivity, so be sure you want a quiet evening!
- Eat a light dinner for improved control over body weight.

DON'T:

- Eat heavy meals, fried foods, or very high-fiber meals, all of which can keep your digestion system churning into the wee hours.
- Eat large amounts of high-protein foods, which may keep you awake.
- Eat foods to which you have a partial intolerance, such as wheat, soy, or dairy products. While well tolerated for breakfast, these foods may make you feel uncomfortable if eaten later in the day.

Bedtime snack

I like to go to bed on an empty stomach. But if you're one of those people who wants to eat before sleeping, here are some tips.

DO:

- Eat slow-release carbs.
- If you're going to have a mini-meal, do eat a small "balanced" snack with both healthy carbs and a small amount of protein, e.g., beans and wild rice.

DON'T

- Eat fast-release carbs, which are worst for you at night when you're not moving and are likely to gain weight. No one likes a short-acting sleeping pill that knocks you out but leaves you staring at the ceiling at 3:00 A.M., which is exactly what can happen if your blood sugar drops precipitously during sleep.
- Don't eat pure protein, which will keep you awake.

Grazing versus Three Squares

In the days when there wasn't much food, large meals evolved as a way of eating as much food as possible after hunting down a large animal or winning another such prehistoric food lottery. Our bodies then went into deep storage mode as a way of holding on to every last calorie until another such highly unpredictable food treasure presented itself. Storage mode means putting on lots of fat, stealing blood flow away from other vital organs, and becoming very lethargic. Large meals were reinstituted during the Industrial Revolution as a way of standardizing mealtimes for maximum worker productivity. We know now that it is better to keep blood glucose level rather than having a daylong boom-and-bust series of cycles. There are two ways to avoid these cycles. One is to eat lean meals that are low in fat, high in protein, and high in soluble fiber foods such as beans. This provides hourslong satiety and a steady blood sugar level if you want to stay with the three-meal-a-day plan. The other strategy is to eat smaller, more frequent meals . . . the emphasis being on meals, not snacks. That means a combination of protein and slow-release carbs, not a bag of pretzels, which will spike your blood sugar and make you drowsy.

Travel

I travel a lot. For instance, in the spring of 1997, I spent a month in the Congo followed by three weeks on a book tour in a different city every day. For *Dateline NBC* I can travel two to three weeks a month. When I first began traveling for *Dateline* I quickly saw how it could tear you apart: lots of missed connections, late flights, late nights, all-night shoots, long drives. I noticed from the start that I was exhausted all the time. I kept up my exercise, but I tried, as I knew I shouldn't have, to compensate for my dip in energy by overeating. Now the tough thing about traveling and doing TV is that you need to look really good and sound sharp at all times . . . no excuses. What I quickly found was that the sugary-food, over-eating, caffeine route failed miserably. I was tired and nervous on camera. It just didn't work. What I fortunately discovered almost immediately, was that a vegetarian program with a little fish made it all work and work well. First, it brought an immediate sense of calm. Second, it drained away the fatigue. Third, my performance improved dramatically. Sure, the nervous energy was gone, but the quiet energy was there in abundance. Boy, what a miracle. I now order vegetarian meals on all flights. I have found all the best natural food markets in America and I've found how to get really quick items that are still superhealthy. Most critically, I found that the sense of calm pervaded to the point that I could get a terrific night's sleep in any hotel. And rather than gaining weight on a trip, I could actually lose it. I had boundless energy to conduct interviews, work out, and still research new pieces and . . . this book!

More than any other diet I know of, the low-glucose, vegetarian diet with a little fish delivers calming effects rarely beaten by even the most powerful drugs — and unlike the drugs, the diet is without harmful, long-lasting side effects. It gives you the ultimate mood control, especially control over anxiety and the "crashing" phenomenon often experienced shortly after food intake. You'll find the healthiest cuisines to be the East Asian, Mediterranean, and Mexican "Sonoran" cuisines. The most practical high-performance work diet is pretty close to a caveman diet . . . that is, it is high in protein, fruits, and vegetables, with few grains for the working day.

Step 5:
Play Hard

———

In our never-ending quest to keep a steady job and pay the mortgage, we lose sight of what life's all about: Life should be a kick. We work incredibly hard, but our play is often dull: reading on a beach, sitting on a luxury liner poop deck, lining up with teeming millions at theme parks. We come back from what's supposed to be a vacation exhausted from too much drink, too much food, and not enough activity. No form of mental dullness is harder to shake than that of the lethargy brought on by all work and no play, or the wrong kind of play. Play should rejuvenate the brain, allowing us to reach for fresh new ideas. A case in point. I was languishing in New York looking for a new book idea. Instead of giving up, I took a working holiday helicopter skiing in British Columbia. No more than 20,000 feet of freshly skied vertical powder later, and the idea for this book came to life. I skied hard all morning and wrote hard all afternoon. By the end of the week, I had an outline in hand.

> **CONVENTIONAL WISDOM:** Be careful, play safe!
> **THE BIOLOGY OF SUCCESS:** If it's not risky, it's
>   not fun.

OK OK OK! Don't kill yourself — risk doesn't mean danger. The point is that what you're doing should provide some challenge and thrill.

The Biology of Playing Hard

In the "brain reward site" that leads to overall well-being, there is an array of neurotransmitters involved in four neurotransmitter pathways: the serotonin, opioid peptides (endorphins), gamma amino butyric acid, and catecholamines (dopamine, noreipephrine) pathways. The area considered to be the primary "reward site" is the nucleus accumbens, says Dr. Kenneth Blum, Adjunct Research Professor in the Department of Biological Science at the University of North Texas and Scientific Director of the Path Medical Foundation in New York. He describes the final sense of reward as the end result of a finely tuned "cascade" of these neurotransmitters, all of which have to work perfectly and in concert for you to feel good. At the very end of this cascade, the neurotransmitter dopamine is released at the nucleus accumbens, and that makes you feel good. Dopamine works by interacting with five dopamine receptors or nerve cell sites, of which the dopamine D-2 receptor is the most important. Dr. Blum and his associates discovered a specific genetic variant associated with low dopamine D-2 receptors. Carriers of this gene have fewer dopamine D-2 receptors and as a result hypo (lower) dopamine function. Dr. Blum has termed this common genetic hypodopaminergic (reduced dopamine D-2 receptors) trait the "Reward Deficiency Syndrome" — it causes a breakdown in the normal workings of our brain's "reward cascade." Dr. Blum and his associates found that one-third of all Americans carry the gene for hypodopamine function! Since everyone needs dopamine for its pleasure- and antistress-inducing qualities, people with "Reward Deficiency Syndrome" often seek out unhealthy addictive substances and behaviors that are known to activate or stimulate nerve cell dopamine release. These substances and behaviors may include alcohol, cocaine, heroin, nicotine, glucose, pathological gambling, addictive sexual activity, or pathological violence. Since dopamine is the neurotransmitter responsible for hands-punched-into-the-sky elation, I am suggesting there is another far safer means of releasing dopamine — learning how to play hard.

For your leisure time, find activities that give you a sense of thrill and challenge. Life should deliver some real forms of elation. In America today we spend an enormous amount of time at the low end of the mood scale. Some psychiatrists even believe that our natural state today is a depressed one. There is too little talk of joy or elation in America today. We have become a depressed and anxious nation. Often it takes a real jolt to bring us back from the precipice. One morning, as a young boy, I was walking home from church, head down, examining every last inch of sidewalk that passed underfoot. My father asked, "Why are you looking down?" "I'm looking for loose change." His response is one I'll never forget. "If you look at the ground you may find a dime, but if you look at the sky, you may get a million-dollar idea."

How to Play Hard

Take up new challenges. Play Walter Mitty. Learn things you've never done before . . . things you've only dreamed of. That could be learning to heli ski, flying a plane, kayaking a raging river, or learning a foreign language or a musical instrument. William F. Buckley says: "I sail, I ski, and I listen to music and play a little harpsichord." A master of understatement, he is a world-class sailor.

When you're choosing an activity that interests and excites you, try to pick something that will pay several dividends — an activity that you love but that will also physiologically raise your mood to a new plane. Sports are a great option, because the exercise component plays such a large role in mood control, and so you are getting a double dividend. Singing is another wonderful option, because it means that you can actively practice your own music therapy. If you sing, lay it all on the line and perform . . . for your family, in a choir, or in a concert. I took opera singing lessons last year; it's the world's best way of improving your speaking voice and a marvelous mood enhancer even though, if you're like me, you'll never want to sing in public. You may find exhilaration by tracking down your genealogical heritage, finding a rare book, or learning about historic treasures — but whatever you choose, look for and find that exhilaration.

A big part of learning well comes from the right kind of instruction. We are turned off from instructors because we often associate them with mean old gym teachers, but when you are footing the bill, you're in charge. Find someone who makes you feel good about yourself. I find talented, thoughtful, and individualized instruction to be wonderful psychotherapy.

If you choose to challenge yourself with an activity that requires intense physical exertion, make sure you're well prepared before you go for the action. What I advocate is judicious risk-taking, not pre-meditated suicide. For some of my friends, action is jumping out of a helicopter onto a snow-capped precipice with skis on, but not jumping off a bridge with a bungee attached! The difference between risk-taking and mere thrill-seeking is that risk-taking is calculated, not mindless. I advocate taking risks, but making certain that you first achieve a very high level of skill to minimize the possibility of accident and maximize your sense of elation when you succeed.

Here's an example of thorough preparation before taking physical risk. Heli skiing sounds like a wildly exotic activity. Yet on my run last year in British Columbia, I was amused to see a group of very ordinary Japanese housewives. They appeared cautious, conservative, and even withdrawn. They were not throwing themselves aimlessly against the mountain. They had spent a week taking powder ski lessons, learning all the right kinds of motions and turns. They rented specialized powder skis. When the moment came to blast off from a steep ridge into bottomless powder, they had the fitness, the equipment, the technique, and the confidence to succeed. Sure, it was a major thrill, but it wasn't mindless and the danger was minimized. At the end of the day, there it was, that look of elation, joy, and accomplishment. Another group I skied with were world-cup surfers from the big island of Hawaii. The surfers had taken up snowboarding and come to British Columbia to ride the ultimate wave, an 11,000-foot virgin peak. The helicopter couldn't fully land on the sharp knife-edged ridge. We just grabbed our gear and steadied ourselves on this precipice as the helicopter hovered. I punched in the *Evita* theme song on my CD player and plunged off the edge onto a 50-degree, 3,000-foot snow-covered wall. When I arrived at the bottom, I looked up to see the surfers on their boards plummet off the edge with a great white plume of fresh powder snow behind them. Wow, I thought, THAT is truly cool.

Lest you think that all action thrills are dedicated to the pursuit of mindless pleasure, consider this. The most vibrant, interesting, and accomplished people I know are in the business of international relief. It is an enormous risk-taking venture. Take, as an example, a flight I took with Americares from JFK to the Congo during the height of the Rwanda refugee crisis. First there were the logistics, organizing an airplane, being certain that the right lifesaving medicines and foods were aboard, obtaining a maze of international overflight clearances . . . all against a drop-dead timeline. Then there was the risk of flying into a highly unstable area. There were French soldiers, mass murders, a rebel force, and a heavily armed and angry government. Yet the final thrill of hitting the ground and getting the much-needed supplies to some of the millions of refugees equaled any sports success you can imagine. Clearly these dedicated professionals hadn't done it for the thrill, but it was there for the taking nonetheless.

You might not want obvious physical risk such as skiing out of a helicopter or skydiving. Risk-taking and its accompanying reward come in all sizes and forms. Doing amateur stand-up comedy, or deciding to get married, or taking singing lessons can all be risks that get your system pumped and thrilled. What you consider risk-taking depends on what you regard as challenging and a bit scary but also thrilling to do . . . and that can be almost anything.

If you're not achieving success in your career, it's doubly important that you feel success in sports, music, art, a hobby, ANYTHING. As a junior high school student, I really struggled. Being in a hotly competitive academic environment, I really felt left behind. But I experienced tremendous success playing the trumpet. In two years I was first trumpet in the New England Conservatory Orchestra. That feeling of success stayed with me my whole life and translated into other success because I'd had a taste of it. My closest friends growing up were champion oarsmen and figure skaters. Their discipline and success on the ice and the water translated into great academic success. When you play hard, you'll experience the real highs in life, so you know what to aim for in your professional, social, and family life. The success you experience while playing hard will lend new vigor and elation to your work and social life and will give you the confidence and optimism to succeed in your life's work.

Step 6:
Get Breathless

——————— |||||| ———————

The hill climbed for ten miles and two thousand vertical feet over the California coastal range. Just in front of me on their bikes were world champion oarsman Rick Grogan, Olympic oarsman Dick Cashin, and seven-time world speed-skiing champion Franz Weber. My heart rate ticked over at 174, with alarm bells buzzing. I was breathing so fast, so deep, and so hard, the group mercifully nicknamed me the "chainsaw" for the noise. My Litespeed titanium Vortex bike creaked and groaned to and fro as I pushed to the biggest gear I could muster. The group began to slip away. I dug down deeper and deeper to find that last bit of resolve to push, to keep up, even though I was at my limit. Not for you? The trouble with exercise is that we in the medical community endlessly pander to the public: less is more, just walk to the bus, everything in moderation. Don't fool yourself. When it comes to success, when it comes to creating mental energy, when it comes to motivation, the very fittest are the very best. Now, that doesn't mean you have to win at sports. I fell off the back of the pack, arriving at the top of the hill minutes after the others. But it didn't matter. I had done the best my physiology allowed me to do. I felt great, the best I had in years. Over time, I too had become a victim of my own pandering . . . running a moderately high heart rate, but never very high, taking it easy, cutting down on excess mileage. But day in day out, up to 120 miles and eight thousand vertical feet a day down the coast of California, I pegged my heart rate at max. What a difference. I resolved, once again, to have the self-discipline to be the very best I could be — a new dimension in mental energy and overall well-being as well as drive.

CONVENTIONAL WISDOM: A little exercise goes a long way.
THE BIOLOGY OF SUCCESS: The harder the better.

The Biology of Activity

Exercise is the magic bullet for creating mental energy. The immediate effect of exercise is increased energy, so tactically it can be used at any point of a flagging day to get you up and going. Regular exercise elevates your overall month-to-month mood and feeling of optimism. Finally, exercise is the single best method available for decreasing the tension and stress that rob you of mental energy. Here's a close look at how exercise changes your biology.

The hormones adrenaline, nonadrenaline, and cortisol all rise with regular exercise. During depression, levels of these hormones decrease, which led researchers to conclude that these hormones are instrumental in the positive effect of exercise on mood. Exercise also increases the brain blood flow, thus allowing more oxygen into the brain, which is key to improving mental energy, especially after waking in the morning or after an afternoon nap. When you are feeling down, exercise improves self-esteem and distracts you from your problems, so you can relax and think more clearly. There is even a euphoria attached to exercise, claim runners who extol the "high." Many studies have linked the positive mood resulting from exercise to endorphin production, though final proof is still lacking. Tom Murphy, longtime Chairman of the ABC Television Network, uses exercise to maintain his energy and success: "I've always exercised. I played squash at lunch or I'd sneak off and swim during lunch. I played squash for half an hour; I'd swim for twenty minutes. I'd always exercise either during lunch or after work, at 6:00 P.M. or 6:30 P.M."

How to Increase Mental Energy with Exercise

For success, there is a tactical (rescuing a day that's going badly) and a strategic (long-term improvement) use of exercise.

Tactical (short-term) energy booster

Researchers have found that one bout of exercise can shift our current psychological state from a foul mood toward a far more positive one. What's more, this positive shift may last for several hours after the exercise has ceased. If I've landed after an overnight flight and gone straight to work, I'll recover by blasting through an hour on the stair machine. The important fact to consider is that psychological states can turn on a dime. A "state" is best demonstrated in a sudden burst of anxiety, as with a close call. Imagine driving your car along a quiet and picturesque dirt road. Your current psychological state is one of relaxation or calm. Now, if a deer appears out of nowhere and causes you to swerve, your mood state is instantly altered to one of anxiety — fear of hitting the animal. Once you are safely past the deer, your psychological state shifts yet again, as relief settles since you got through the close call unscathed. This probably all occurred within less than a minute. Rather than being held captive to the psychological turns of the day, consider that you can choose to alter dramatically your mood. For example, when you're in a high-stress, high-anxiety situation, a high-intensity workout of twenty or more minutes will calm you down.

Dr. John Silber, who was President of Boston University from 1971 to 1996, has long believed in the tactical use of exercise: "I like to swim, but I don't have a pool in my backyard. I have a treadmill and bicycle and five-pound weights, and I use these almost every day. I start with situps, then weights. Then I get on the treadmill for twenty minutes. I bring my heartbeat to 150–160 beats; and then I do four minutes of biking. Thirty minutes, all in all. I find that exercising generates energy. If you feel dull and in need of sleep, exercise instead. By the time you're done exercising you'll feel energized."

Strategic (long-term) energy enhancement

As adults, few of us actually believe that we can change much if anything of our personality, because traits are considered permanent parts of our established personality. That's why it's all the more amazing to find you can actually change personality traits. When subjects adopt a long-term exercise program, they *do* change their psychological traits, as evidenced by long-term psychological profiles. That's the good news. The bad news is that psychological traits are rarely affected by a single bout of exercise; rather, they change with regular daily activity. I swear the only reason that many of my friends and I are upbeat at all is that we have great exercise programs. In all studies done on daily mood alone (not depression or anxiety), researchers found an improvement in mood after exercise trials.

Mood Effects

Foul-mood immunity

William Morgan, Ed.D., a professor in the Department of Kinesiology at the University of Wisconsin–Madison, says the overwhelming consensus is that the better the physical fitness, the better the mental health! Exercise wards off depression, anxiety, and other affective disorders. For patients with moderate anxiety and depression, a regular exercise program (strength, flexibility, or cardiovascular) is as beneficial as standard forms of psychological counseling. Some animal studies suggest that exercise can modify brain neurotransmitters in the same way that antidepressant drugs do.

Depression

Now, for the first time, researchers are monitoring the long-term reduction of depressive symptoms using only exercise, instead of pharmaceutical treatment. Most people suffering from depression are easily treated, and exercise is now becoming recognized as an alternative to pharmaceuticals and psychotherapy — with fewer side effects and lower cost. At the Cooper Institute for Aerobics

Research, in Dallas, Texas, a study is under way to examine the effect of different doses of exercise as a sole treatment for mild to moderate depression. According to Michael Norden, M.D., author of *Beyond Prozac* and a practicing psychiatrist in Seattle, Washington, exercise has a clearly established ability to raise serotonin. He says, "Ninety minutes on a treadmill doubles brain serotonin levels."

Anxiety

Contrary to traditional belief that patients with anxiety disorders should not exercise vigorously lest they experience a panic attack, recent studies indicate that patients with anxiety disorders who are free of physical disorders (e.g., mitral valve prolapse) would actually benefit psychologically from an exercise program.

Stress

There is good evidence to show that exercise is an effective stress reliever, and that many people use exercise precisely to relieve stress.

Self-image

Even in your late thirties or early forties you may start feeling the slow creep of advancing age. The kids seem to be passing you by; you look different to yourself. That can take a big chip out of your self-esteem. I have found no better means of fighting time than by actually *being* younger. David Costill, professor of exercise physiology at Ball State University, has consistently shown that a fit fifty-year-old could have far more physical prowess, measured as muscle strength and aerobic conditioning, than a sedentary twenty-five-year-old. Even more amazing is that you can retain the aerobic prowess of a twenty-one-year-old into your fifties.

Practical Guide to Exercise

Choosing an exercise

Steady rhythmic exercise with little impact — for example, walking, biking, rowing, cross-country skiing, hiking and stair climbing — gives you immediate energy. I find the best exercises are the ones that I can do the longest and hardest. For that reason I like exercises that can offer a minimum load on the bones, joints, and ligaments yet a maximum impact on major muscle groups. Cycling is a perfect example. On a bike you can almost go forever. More practically, you can cruise along in a trance for hours at a time, yet you can also suddenly hammer at high intensity with little of the risk of injury found in high-impact sports such as aerobic dance. Stair machines, cross-country ski machines, spinning machines, and treadmills are the twenty-first-century tranquilizer. Nearly always available, they're a great stress breaker in the middle of the day and a great way to pick up energy in the mid to late afternoon.

If your major occupation makes you aggressive or even belligerent, you might want to take up boxing as an exercise and outlet for recovery. Or you might be in a job or a career that requires you to fight for what is right! When you really need to get angry, very intensive exercise brings on the mental power and determination to get the job done. When I'm facing a really tough issue, I'll go on a long, high-intensity workout and get pumped to settle the issue.

Intensity

I find vigorous exercise far more effective than moderate exercise for lowering my tension level for the rest of the day. Vigorous exercise is also the best way to control your weight, because it puts your body into a fat-burning phase for several hours after the workout. Since most of us are not highly trained professional athletes, continuous high-intensity exercise is tough to do. Intervals are the best alternative.

Intervals

Long the preserve of elite-class athletes, intervals are the biggest secret in training today. Nothing but nothing will change your mood faster. Intervals offer a way to dramatically burn off anxiety and stress in a short period of time. Intervals are performed by going all out for short periods of time. I like one- to two-minute periods "on" at high intensity followed by a low intensity for several minutes. This builds speed, power, and a great mood without the need to go all out for long periods of time. Intervals undertaken as part of an aerobic workout have another key advantage: They are the best way of burning large amounts of fat after your workout. Research shows that after a high-intensity workout, fat burning increases to its highest capacity and continues to do so for hours. Slip away from the office to the gym for just twenty minutes on a stair machine. Even if you're tired, you can still punch out ten good one-minute intervals. I also love intervals as a way of jump-starting my metabolism. This is great when fighting jet lag. Spin classes, stair machines, and bikes are great ways of doing interval training without running the risk of injury. One important note: Intervals do require strong ligaments, tendons, joints, and muscles. That means you'll want to have a good "base" of training before attempting intervals. Training assures that your body is "hardened" against injury. Since your heart is your most important muscle, check with your doctor before you consider intervals, and inquire about exercise stress testing if you're over fifty or at risk for heart disease.

Deep breathing

In a study published in 1992, Bonnie G. Berger and David R. Owen of Brooklyn College compared mood benefits of different types of exercise and found that what is important may be the abdominal breathing and not the aerobic component of exercise. They reported that "stress-reduction benefits of Hatha yoga were similar to those previously reported for jogging and swimming."* Hatha yoga is the physical exercise form of yoga; it emphasizes various body positions or asanas entailing balancing, stretching, and breathing routines that help increase your flexibility and static muscle. Using Hatha yoga, participants strengthen and relax major muscle groups that may have contracted as a result of stress or faulty posture. In Berger and Owen's study, Hatha yoga met seven of the eight stress-reducing criteria with the exception of aerobic exercise. Swimming, on the other hand, met all eight of the requirements. Both swimmers and Hatha yoga participants reported significant short-term benefits and decreases in anger, confusion, tension, and depression. Since Hatha yoga is not an aerobic exercise, Berger and Owen

---

*Bonnie G. Berger and David R. Owen, "Mood Alteration with Yoga and Swimming: Aerobic Exercise May Not Be Necessary," *Perceptual and Motor Skills* 75 (1992): 1333.

concluded that it was the abdominal breathing, not the aerobic component, that was beneficial. The rhythmical diaphragmatic breathing that yoga incorporates is also a by-product of the aerobic training that facilitates mood alteration; so rather than being simply aerobic, exercise should promote the kind of controlled abdominal breathing common to several meditation techniques as well. I've settled on Qigong, an ancient Chinese healing art. It combines prolonged deep breathing, long slow movements of the arm and body, and meditation. I practice Qigong waiting in lines at the airport, when trying to fall asleep in a strange setting, before a major interview, anywhere I need to relax. I found it a wonderful energy builder at any time of day, producing the ideal state: calm energy. I learned it at The Land of Medicine Buddha in Santa Cruz, California. Instructional classes are available in most major cities. You can pick up enough in a day or two to get a great deal out of Qigong quite quickly.

Weight training

As a middle-of-the day stress buster, weight training is terrific. Weight training is especially good for cutting the effect of stress on the neck and shoulders. For that reason, exercises that affect the deltoids and trapezius go a long way to building up resistance to stress. The best stress-busting routines and the ones that make you feel hard and toned are with moderate resistance, 12–18 repetitions. Be sure to squeeze the last two reps so you get a real burn. By avoiding very high resistance, you'll experience less muscle soreness and a greater feeling of well-being. I like to do a series of deep breathing exercises during weight training to push my breathing just as I would on a fast run or bike ride. Try alternating a set of triceps dips with a set of pull-ups to push your breathing even harder. The complete set of weight training exercises is available in my book *Turning Back the Clock*.

How much

Benefits just keep increasing as you increase the length and intensity of the workout. Some experts believe that in order to reap the full health benefits of exercise, you will need to exercise vigorously for four hours every week. You might ask, "How much exactly is the much-talked-about moderate intensity? Can you give me a figure?" Whether you choose a medium- or high-fitness-level program, you will need to understand what each category means. Fitness is a continuous variable — we can talk about high, very high, extremely high fitness, and so on, but I think we can make the following distinctions:

MODERATE FITNESS

If you run a few miles several times a week, you're moderately fit. Thirty minutes of brisk walking will also get you out of the low-fit and into the moderately-fit category. Brisk walking means being able to walk one mile in 15–20 minutes. A well-balanced moderate fitness program would include at minimum: (a) thirty minutes of brisk walking every day — you can accumulate that in three ten-minute walks — and (b) two or three times a week some weight lifting and stretching, or other activities that condition the muscles.

HIGH FITNESS

To be highly fit, you have to exercise more than thirty minutes a day every day — this could mean running/jogging for thirty or more minutes, or doing moderate-level exercise for more than thirty minutes every day. Dr. Steven Blair of the Cooper Institute for Aerobics Research says that running anywhere from 20 to 50 miles a week would put you in the highly fit category. Even at 40–50 miles a week, there is no increased risk of premature mortality, although people who run that much are more likely to experience bone and joint injuries and may also be more likely to impair immune function. If you'd rather bike, blade, cross-country ski, swim, hike, or power walk, then for high fitness you would need up to an hour of vigorous exercise per day.

If you're going for more than moderate fitness, be sure to get a good evaluation and recommendations from an orthopedic surgeon who practices sports medicine to be sure you aren't going to damage ligaments, joints, or tendons by going too hard or too fast.

And if you have risk factors for heart disease or are over fifty, be sure to consult your cardiologist before undertaking any rigorous exercise programs.

Exercise environment

Always wondered why it's harder to exercise indoors? Jane Harte and George Eifert's study found that the group that exercised outdoors had the most positive moods during and following exercise, while those who exercised indoors and had no external stimuli showed the least positive affect, and, in fact, showed a negative mood following the exercise bout.* Harte and Eifert noted that runners who exercised indoors with no external stimuli naturally focused on the actual exercise and their bodies' response to it; the runners noticed their own heavy breathing and maybe some accompanying discomfort. The act of exercise became tedious, and the bout of exercise was shorter, resulting in negative mood. The environment even affected the runners' biology: indoor and outdoor runners showed different patterns of urinary adrenaline, noradrenaline, and cortisol excretion. In their study on swimming and yoga, Bonnie G. Berger and David R. Owen also found that uncomfortable exercise surroundings can actually have a negative effect on mood; when swimmers exercised in a too-warm water temperature of 106°F, their mood became negative. If you have to exercise indoors, as many of us do, you can still boost your mood by exercising with a class, boosting your spirits with music, or finding a gym with lots of windows facing onto the great outdoors.

Overdoing it

The biggest scam in exercise today is the chorus of voices warning against overexercise. We're the most overweight, unfit nation on the face of the planet. Only 12 percent of us are exercising at the level suggested by the American College of Sports Medicine Exercise

---

*Jane L. Harte and George H. Eifert, "The Effect of Running, Environment, and Attentional Focus on Athletes' Catecholamine and Cortisol Levels and Mood," in *Psychophysiology* 32 (1995): 49–54.

Prescription. How many of us overtrain? Less than one-tenth of 1 percent, guesses Dr. Andrea Dunn of the Cooper Institute for Aerobics Research. If you're in that one-tenth of 1 percent, exercise can backfire — "when top athletes are overtrained, they start having symptoms similar to clinical depression," says Dr. Dunn. Yuri Hanin, Ph.D., professor and senior researcher at the Research Institute for Olympic Sports in Finland, says that if exercise is of a very high intensity, there is a rise in anxiety during the workout. Here's why. During intensive exercise, when positive affect has been depleted and resources are limited, athletes sometimes resort to negative affect for energy resources to keep going. For example, Professor Hanin found that at the end of 50-kilometer ski races, the athlete is shifting and postponing and fighting fatigue, and generates or recruits negative emotions to finish. Long-distance runners, bike racers, and triathletes may experience a similar negative mood shift at the end of the race. I've found that whereas a 10-kilometer road race, 40-mile bike race, or short course triathlon may boost my mood, a marathon, 100-mile bike race, or iron-man contest may lower it. That's in part why I now opt for the shorter races. Professor Hanin's explanation is that some emotions, such as anger, tension, or dissatisfaction, are energizing, while others, such as contentment, are not. But remember, Professor Hanin was examining professional athletes who were running 50-kilometer races. If you've gotten that far in your fitness, congratulations! You have the fitness to control your moods, to generate any emotion you need when you need it! For most of us not running 50-kilometer races, intense exercise can be a great place to work through negative emotions so we feel more terrific afterward. Whether you're reaching down for the motivation to begin a program or pushing for the next level of fitness, remember that the more fitness becomes part of your success, the more you will want to embrace it.

Step 7: Look Like
a Star

OK, sure, this is the decade of dress down, but ask yourself honestly: Do you really feel great if you dress down or do you feel less than your best? I can remember standing in the Iraqi desert with a group of refugees from Bangladesh. These poor people had lost everything they ever hoped for — their homes, jobs, money, family. They were stranded in the desert after Saddam Hussein invaded Kuwait and drove them out. Yet each and every one of them was superbly groomed. They were fresh, crisp, clean shaven, with immaculate clothes. Now you may think that's a waste of time. But the first sign of a lack in self-esteem is dressing down. Taking the time and effort to dress well has a marked daily effect on mood. That's why the ritual of dressing, shaving, or applying makeup, and choosing your clothes with care can make a big difference. So concentrate and enjoy your morning grooming; it's therapeutic, not a waste of time.

> **CONVENTIONAL WISDOM:** Clothes make the man.
>
> **THE BIOLOGY OF SUCCESS:** Appearance creates self-esteem, which breeds success.

Freud himself said that physical pleasure was not an end itself but a means to building and enhancing self-esteem, David Keirsey reminds us in his excellent book *Please Understand Me*. For certain temperaments, a sense of pleasure in surroundings, clothing, and general celebration of daily life allows them to think more highly of themselves. We looked carefully at creating a prized space around you in your work environment. Now let's look at clothing as a way of taking that space with you.

Dress

Do you ever say, "Well, nothing important will happen today, so I'll just wear a wrinkled old pair of pants and yesterday's shirt"? How many times have you done that only to find yourself in an extremely important meeting? But even more important is the concept that if you dress down you've decided that nothing important will happen. Companies that use Friday as a dress-down day have ensured that nothing important will happen on that day.

In life there are very few things that we have real control over. One of them is our appearance. This may really seem trivial, but the truth is that every time we let our appearance go we are letting go an opportunity to control our fate . . . we are giving in to pessimism. Those Bangladesh refugees who made such a great impression on worldwide television news soon received treatment accorded to none of the other refugees. They were picked up by a giant Russian Antonov aircraft and flown home.

Even if by nature you're a very modest person, put in a good appearance. Mother Teresa may have worn simple clothes, but she always looked like a star, and so should you.

Always try to be appropriately dressed so that you're transmitting a consistent message. You don't want to look one way and speak another, or feel one way and look another. A psychiatrist friend of mine told me about a thirty-nine-year-old patient he had. The woman had badly bleached hair, poorly applied makeup, and clothes that could only be described as sleazy. She complained to him of one abusive relationship after another. The psychiatrist desperately wanted to say: Get a grip, look at yourself in the mirror. Professional standards prevented him from doing so. The woman then decided to take a motivational course. The instructor, before he even addressed the audience in general, looked down at this woman and said, "You look like a hooker. Look at your makeup. It's terrible. Your hair's a wreck and your clothes look like a hooker's." Even though the story seems incredibly sexist, the woman took the message to heart. She had her hair professionally colored. She learned to apply a subtle form of makeup. She bought sophisticated new clothes. She was transformed. Her relationships improved. She got new and better employment. She learned that she needed to impress herself as much as anyone else.

Style

Ralph Lauren has built the largest fashion business in the history of fashion. His message is simple: There is a distinction between fashion and style; style is related to the person and is more enduring whereas fashion is more related to the times. If you want to be fashionable, you just go out and buy what's in vogue, but that will not endure. If you're going to derive real satisfaction and confidence from your clothing, you'll want to develop your own style. So look at yourself, look at your clothes, and dress for success.

Matching Your Biology to Your Dress

The key is matching your clothing to your physique. "Dressing well is much like building a house. You need the proper foundation to build the house," says Alan Flusser. Alan designed Michael Douglas's clothes for the film *Wall Street*, and has sold more books on clothing that anyone else (he is author of *Style and the Man, Clothes and the Man,* and *Shopping around the World*). Alan teaches men how to wear a suit, shirt, tie, socks, shoes, and handkerchief that suit their physique. If you can do that, then you have the basis for building a personal style that can transcend the vagaries of fashion. "Ninety-eight percent of the fashion-buying public does not know how to do that," Alan says. Whether men or women, "they don't know the correct jacket length for their torso, correct sleeve length, or correct shirt-collar design for their face, just for starters." And yet, Alan points out, in the last twenty years, men have spent more on clothes than in the history of this century. Dressing well can be incredibly easy, Alan says, and you only have to learn it once. Alan offers the following general guidelines, and although he works with men's clothing, he thinks these tips are useful to women as well.

Your face

Your clothes should lead the viewer's eye toward your face. You don't want to have the colors or proportion of the clothes compete or distract from the most important communicator, which is your face. On the other hand, you want to wear and choose clothes that present your face in its most healthy form. Clothes are about framing and presenting the face in color and in proportion.

Color

You want the colors of your clothes to harmonize with and enliven your face, not to detract from it. Rather than sticking to a particular color, try to understand the color scheme that suits you best. People can be typed according to one of two general color concepts: either they have contrast, or they are muted. First ascertain this, and then, when trying to harmonize colors with your complexion, realize that the harmony itself can be of contrast or muted.

"CONTRAST PEOPLE"

- Contrast people have contrast between their skin and hair color. For example, they might have very dark hair and very fair skin.

- Contrast people should wear colors that contrast with one another and with the skin color. They need strong color to support their complexion; weak colors would dilute the natural strength in the face.

- If you are a contrast person and you wear muted colors underneath your chin, the colors will not highlight the natural contrast that exists in your face, and that will deaden your appearance; your skin will not be as alive or brilliant as when the colors that are surrounding it are in contrast with one another and/or with your face.

- Example: Al Gore has high contrast, and looks good in dark suits, white shirts, and a dark tie.

"MUTED PEOPLE"

- Muted people do not have much contrast between their skin and hair color. For example, they might have blond hair and fair skin.

- Muted people should wear colors that don't contrast with one another and with the skin.

- If you have muted colors and you wear a high-contrast combination of colors, you will overwhelm or distract from the less strong or muted colors of your visage.

- Example: Bill Gates has muted colors; he does not have much contrast between hair and skin color and consequently looks best in colors that don't contrast with one another — for example a blue rather than a white shirt with a dark suit.

MORE TIPS ON COLOR

- Once you've determined whether you have contrast or are muted, you can make more subtle judgments. Are you a person of high or low contrast? Do you have blue or brown eyes? Do you have freckles? As you answer such questions you'll be able to make more sophisticated decisions about the level of contrast in the color schemes you choose.

- Unless they have very high contrast, most men look best in a blue shirt, because it doesn't drain their face of color as a white shirt would. Notice how when men go on TV they are encouraged to wear blue shirts — the lighting and camera make the face less sallow with a blue shirt than with a white one. You can't make such a generalization about women because women wear makeup which could change the contrast and add a whole new dimension to the face.

- When you choose a color, put it up against your face.

Proportion

Proportion is the key to dressing well and the main criterion of longevity. "If I had to choose proportion or color, I would choose proportion," says Alan Flusser. For example, if a man asks for a custom-tailored blue blazer that is too long and that has shoulders that are too broad, he won't look his best in it, and he'll soon throw it out. For both men and women, if the proportions of your clothes are right, you can carry off a wider variety of experimental colors and patterns. Basically, people tend to look good in one or two kinds of proportions, not four or five.

If you saw a man or woman dressed in clothes of the right proportion, he or she would look great, even if the actual clothes were of poor quality. Knowledge of the correct proportions relative to your own physique is not illusionary; it's finite, and a tailor will help you understand it. You need to have and apply the correct information. Unless you have exactly the same proportions as the model used to make the clothes, you'll need to have your clothes tailored a little so that they fit perfectly.

Dressing well is not a function of how much you spend. You can spend little and be well dressed, or spend a fortune and be terribly dressed. In addition to color, proportion, and cost, you should consider the fabric of your clothes. You'll also want to pay great attention to your shoes, handbags (for women), neckwear (for men), and accessories such as jewelry, belts, handkerchiefs, or scarves.

The best-dressed people pick one or two silhouettes of clothing and stick with it. They never wear one look one day and another the next day. They buy clothes that can fit together; they concentrate on color range and proportion, so that one can go with the other. Simple in cut and pattern is usually best. Diana Vreeland, the famous *Vogue* editor, would always wear gray/charcoal colors, good shoes, and a red accent . . . and she was always considered extremely chic. The more sophisticated your taste becomes, the more you'll know what looks best on you.

Dressing is an art form. You have to take the time to learn what's appropriate for you and what's not; that may fly in the face of what the current fashion proposes.

Dressing for Success

Clothes are a language, and because they're an illustrative form of expression, you can use them strategically in your career. For people who understand how to use them, clothes are one of the strongest forms of communication. You might have only one chance to make a lasting impression . . . and clothes can be a major aid in getting you in the door and having people give you an opportunity. It would be irresponsible to blow that opportunity by dressing inappropriately. If you're being hired as a computer hunk, then it won't matter what you're wearing, but if you're going to be in a position of selling anything, presentation is what it's all about, and even if you're not perfectly qualified, with the right clothing you'll have a better shot at convincing someone to take a chance on you. The bestselling book in the history of books about men's clothes and the social phenomenon of dress is John Molloy's *Dress for Success.* And John Molloy's simple message is that there is a relationship between how you dress and your level of success. You have to dress for success. Molloy's suggestions range from the sensible advice that if you wear a suit to an interview, you'll be considered more seriously, to the more absurd suggestion that if in the corporate world your boss wears his handkerchief upside down, then you too should wear yours upside down! When you go in for an interview, you've usually researched the company so that you're familiar with its business ways, plans, objectives, and so on. Now make it a point also to research the company's dress culture.

Even without your noticing it, your clothes are already saying much. They're telling about your background, your culture, your social upbringing, schooling, taste, level of sophistication, and, perhaps most importantly . . . they're speaking volumes about how you feel about yourself and your life.

Of course clothes are not a substitute to developing your inner life, but they can give you tremendous confidence and boost your self-esteem. Every time you choose to put something on, you're saying something about yourself. Since much of self-esteem comes from your perception of how others view you, if you get up and put on clothes that you feel look good, it can give you tremendous confidence to take on the day. And this confidence will translate into better work — if you feel good in your clothes you'll have an additional lift to help you become more effective in your day-to-day life.

Step 8:
Set a Ritual

———— ⊪⊪⊪⊪ ————

It's 10:22 A.M. You're on your cell phone, racing down an escalator in an office building in the heart of Manhattan. Once outside, you dive through the crowds, braving a driving rain storm to hail a cab. Determined to beat midtown gridlock, you furiously bark orders at your driver, who is doing his best to duck and weave through traffic. Your secretary calls ahead to flight operations in a desperate attempt to hold on to your seat while you punch one number after the other into your cell phone. At 10:56 you arrive at the airport, spring past scores of fellow travelers, jump the line at security, and race to the gate. It's 10:59:47. Congratulations! You've made the 11:00 shuttle to Boston. You're a hero! Or are you? What have you done? You've caught an airplane. Something millions of people around the world successfully accomplish every day. You've haven't won a war, captured public enemy number one, been elected president, or won the Nobel Prize. You just caught a plane. You performed what should have been a simple ritual of everyday life, yet it consumed your entire being for nearly an hour and left you drained for hours more . . . and it brought out your worst behavior. If you create too much chaos in your life, you can't concentrate on being really creative in your work. I wasted years of my own life doing just that — arriving too late for planes, generating excitement just by making chaos out of the activities of daily living instead of creating excitement in my profession.

Ever wonder what happened to that guy who was the heart of every party? The fellow who ran his life on the ragged edge, racing cars down city streets, drinking until dawn, being disheveled at work? Chances are, in the end, he never made the big time. Why? Many of us confuse lots of craziness in our everyday routines for wildness in our creative lives. To be truly successful, you must follow a ritual. Be as regular as a Swiss clock, ritualize the routines of your everyday life, and you will allow yourself to do what seems impossible: to be wild and exotic in your life's work.

> **CONVENTIONAL WISDOM:** Rituals are for monks.
> **THE BIOLOGY OF SUCCESS:** Rituals are the foun-
> dation of success. Be dull in your everyday rou-
> tines so you can be wildly creative in your work.

The Biology of Rituals

Routines simplify, clarify, and create order, symmetry, and familiarity in chaos and high stress. The human species does not respond well to change, and nowadays the world is changing extremely rapidly and people's lives are in greater flux than ever before. The storms of business and a high-paced life wash away the anchors that create a sense of personal control; and so rituals become doubly important to anchor our time and ensure that what is important in life gets done regardless of how crazy life becomes. Ritual sanctifies time; it places a critical order on a specific activity and elevates it to a preeminent place of importance.

During high stress, rituals are like landing pads in a storm; you come out of the storm and touch on something familiar and then launch back out into storm. If you don't have these landing pads, then the chaos persists. Dr. Jim Loehr, who runs LGE Performance Systems, Inc., a toughening center that trains top athletes, executives, rescue squads, and antiterrorist groups, says that the most accomplished high-stress performers all have defined specific rituals in all areas of their life. "Top performers have lives full of rituals on and off the court. Less accomplished athletes don't have these rituals." Dr. Loehr emphasizes that in every single arena of high stress, whether in sports, the military, medicine, or business, the more demanding the performance, the more people rely on ritual to do the job. Surgeons have precise preoperative routines; pilots have preflight rituals; and at the most basic level, we all have personal hygiene rituals in the morning — think about your morning ritual and how if you skip it, you have a much tougher time launching your day.

Rituals free you to concentrate on what's really important. Once you set them, rituals will save you time because you won't have to plan or think about them; they are automatic, sit in the background, and have a fixed time and place within your day. But rituals are also at the heart of creating brain energy. We've seen how exercise, food, sleep, music, even the proper dress, create mental energy. Rituals first and foremost synchronize our biological clocks with the precision of a fine Swiss timepiece. The surest way to break that synchrony is to disrupt the ritual — you cut short your sleep or sleep at irregular hours, or you don't eat properly, and as a result you mix up glucose and insulin levels and your energy utilization becomes faulty. Both not sleeping and not eating right cause a desynchronization that indicates your behavior is severely affecting your ECP. Creating the biologically successful day is firmly routed in using food, sleep, music, and other activities at the right times of day to get the maximum out of your biological clock. Mark H. McCormack, the very first sports agent, now Chairman and Chief Executive Officer of International Management Group (IMG), the world leader in athlete management and sports marketing, swears by ritual: "I try to be extraordinarily organized and try to compartmentalize my time into dictation, meetings, phone calls, nap, relaxation, and meals."

Stacking for Success

There is a new phenomenon in America called stacking. We all do it. What is stacking? We pile dozens of different tasks one upon the other during any given part of the day. We prepare lunches for our children even as we're feeding them breakfast, calling the plumber, checking our voice mail, and leaving a note for the carpenter. At work, we carry on several running conversations while fielding phone calls, typing a report into a computer, and catching up on required reading. Even while we're telling a bedtime story to our children, we're logging on to check our e-mail yet again and still fielding multiple calls from work. Why do we stack? The conventional explanation is that we have too much to do so we have to perform many tasks simultaneously. The other explanation is that we pile on activities that make us feel good. The right stack of activities manipulates our mood. We open our e-mail, make a phone call, listen to our voice mail all in the expectation that something good has happened or that we will learn something that will surprise us. Simply put, the events of the day can strikingly alter our mood for better or for worse. Many of us already subconsciously stack activities to feel good, but by carefully orchestrating the right stacks of activities at the right times, we can create the perfectly successful day with high mental energy and great efficiency. Don't just pile it on, thinking the more the better. Tactically stack your activities for success.

Strangely enough, it isn't the events themselves that change our mood, it is how they meet our expectations of them. For instance, you could anticipate a spectacular event, a terrific meal at a great restaurant, but the actual meal, while good, doesn't blow you away. It doesn't *exceed* your expectations. The same thing happens with vacations. You've had a ball planning it. Your visions of the trip excite you every time you read more about the destination. Then the big day comes. You take the flight and disembark at East Anguilla. Hey it's a really great place, but it doesn't exceed your expectations, so it doesn't improve your mood. Take a bad event. You go to a friend's funeral. The expectation is that you are going to feel simply terrible. But the sermon is tremendously uplifting, the music is to die for. You leave feeling terrific. Now, those are both life events — a long-planned vacation and a personal tragedy. But every day we anticipate life's smaller turns . . . is the coffee hotter or better tasting than we imagined? Does the newspaper have an amazing article on some far-flung planet in the solar system? No one small incident will make or break your day . . . but as the day goes on the accumulation of these small events might make or break the day depending on how your expectations are met.

Stack too many events that fail to meet your expectations and it won't take much to drag you down into a foul mood . . . the FedEx package that didn't get delivered overnight, the mortgage check that bounces, a phone line that keeps turning up busy. That's why you want to plow into negative stacks when you still feel like a bull, expecting the worst and perhaps being pleasantly surprised. Stack one potentially pleasing event after the other and your mood is buoyed up: a friendly hello, an animated conversation about the weekend, a small tax refund. Of course you can't predict the outcome of all your stacked activities . . . and you wouldn't want to. If *everything* met your expectations, life would be dull. Remember the ad of the aristocratic-looking gentleman in the Rolls-Royce asking the other equally aristocratic-looking gentleman in the other Rolls for the Grey Poupon? Did he look happy? No! In fact, the ad played on our common notion that most rich people don't look happy because they control their environment so tightly that everything meets their expectation but little exceeds it — they look blasé, bored, dull! Do you ask your friends how things are going only to hear "same old, same old"? Pretty boring. Do you wonder why letter carriers go postal? Pretty dull job. Subconsciously, many of us dread predictability and endless repetition, so we become bad stackers. We pile on lots of different activities, hoping, praying that the result will somehow surprise us and exceed our expectations.

Endlessly fishing for a pleasant surprise — lots of phone calls, popping into the hallway in search of a quick conversation, shifting from opening our mail to checking our calendar — all that can make us pretty productive in terms of busywork, but it's not going to lead to the Nobel Prize. Randomly spilling these stacks throughout the day kills our productivity. Mozart didn't write symphonies by making a dozen calls from his cell phone. You need to have concentrated stretches of time when you can focus on the major tasks that make the biggest difference. I call this "prime" time when you perform your most creative work, as opposed to "off-peak" time when you are performing more mundane but still necessary tasks. Too many of us get caught in the trap of remaining in the "off-peak" loop. At day's end, or life's end, we've done a lot, but we can't show major accomplishments. We haven't penned the great American novel or written a hit musical. You may mock such achievements as unrealistic, unrealizable, but in fact many people *do* make the quality time in their lives to accomplish great things.

Intelligently stack both the very important and the not-so-important activities in your life. Learn to use the smaller activities to enhance your mood. For instance, if you're writing a long report during the afternoon, are losing your concentration, and your mood is falling, make a few calls to cheer yourself up. If you know you have some onerous tasks, undertake them while your mood is still high. For instance, make tough phone calls midmorning when you are at the top of your game, not in the late afternoon when you'll be as tough as limp pasta. But don't waste your most precious mental energy on routine phone calls; do your most creative work first, then hit the hard and important calls before the midday crash. The bottom line is that you want to place your stacks in specific time periods during your day.

The aim of strategically placing your stacks is to give yourself stunning mental energy. So prepare ahead for both your more mindless and more mindful activities. Identify, order, and stack your activities . . . and stick to your stacking order. If you have blocked out an hour to write, try to use the entire hour. This is especially difficult in our modern day and age because everything is quick — quick sex, fast food, thirty-second phone calls, and two-minute meetings. If you haven't planned your stacks, it's easier for a few (perhaps even unimportant) mishaps to generate low, negative energy and a terrible mood. For example, three bad phone calls, especially ones late in the afternoon, could put you in a funk, and then you might start looking for other ways of building your mood . . . maybe with alcohol or the wrong kinds of food. Better to short-circuit the downward spiral and plan ahead for a late-afternoon exercise break.

In the end, proper stacking is like being a great deejay, with just the right mix of songs at the right time of day to adjust your mood perfectly. The first step is becoming aware of how your mood does change, then beginning to manipulate it by placing specific stacks of activities at specific times of day. Later in this chapter, in the section titled "How to Create a Ritual," you will find guidelines on how to stack effectively.

First Simplify

Before you develop a stacking order and create your rituals, first simplify your life. When you're simplifying, consider your entire lifestyle and your approach to money. An expensive lifestyle consumes huge amounts of effort — time maintaining homes, boats, cars, and airplanes . . . all time better spent on your life's work. Even shopping can often require more effort than it's worth and can even provoke anxiety . . . especially in men. Too cheap a lifestyle has the same effect. I know businesspeople who spend hours of their day in nearly pointless detail. They'll endlessly negotiate the lowest airfare through connecting cities, then time their watches for the precise minute they can call the airplane for an upgrade. They view trip planning as a creative triumph, but fail to notice that the related stress, anxiety, and time drain is sucking away from their productive time. You could even be wasting your time when you're waiting for a bus instead of just taking a cab from the airport. If you can't afford a cab or your company has already booked you a seat, fine. Sometimes, however, the fight to be cheap eats up a lot more time than it's worth. Consider what your time is worth, then ask if it's worth taking hours of prime time away from your primary job to find the cheapest route or the lowest fare.

Phones, cell phones, pagers, voice mail, e-mail, can all become too much. In this age of technological complexity, simplify your use of electronics. Chances are, whatever your job, you have to deal with some electronics. As a journalist, one can become overwhelmed by electronics. On a recent trip to Albania, during the Kosovo refugee crisis, I packed two computers, an iridium phone, three cell phones, a still camera, portable video camera, pager, dozens of special connectors, chargers, batteries, and wires, extra disks, hard drives, timers, watches, and even a shortwave radio. It has taken me several years to understand that less is more. I used to spend hours each week synchronizing my work computer with my home computer with my travel laptop with my palm pilot. I became like a full-service computer repair station. I'd order all the extra bells and whistles and spend even more hours trying to install them, then wait on hold for customer service to explain their use. Now when I'm traveling in the United States, I vastly simplify my electronic life by having a single computer I use for everything. It's a Macintosh G3 laptop, and I carry it nearly everywhere. Its screen allows me to see two full pages and makes writing books easy and fun even on the road and in airplanes. I save a full working day every two weeks now that I no longer bother with constant updating, upgrading, file swapping, and file syncing. As to the phone, for life on the road in the U.S., I rely on a nationwide one-rate phone. I can get text or voice mail messages sent to it, receive paging, and route all my calls. I can even forward it to a cell phone in seventy foreign countries when I travel. I have two phones for outgoing calls and one for incoming calls. Between the phone and the computer, I'm at the office wherever I am . . . no need to get organized. I'm instantly set up and ready to go. Life's a lot simpler and easier.

How to Create a Ritual

"World-class ritual produces world-class performance," says Dr. Loehr. He and his team create customized rituals that help keep the athletes in sync with their biological clock. Rituals include a set time with family, a set time for a hobby, for eating, exercising, and working. In routing, anchoring, and securing time, ritual is the key element. Ritual means setting a clear routine or time for all routine activities. Plan your week ahead of time, set a schedule, and stick to it. The way to get rituals to work for you is to be certain that you are setting key rituals at a time when they either work best with your biological clock or boost it. In previous chapters, examples included eating or exercising when your rhythms are at a low ebb to boost them, or carefully planning sleep and waking times to boost your clock. Start by establishing great sleep rituals, then add exercise and eating. You'll notice that even these small changes will dramatically improve your prime-time creative activities. As you become more confident in ritual building, carefully partition out more of your day to include time with family, time for hobbies, even time for TV and reading. Setting up your week in advance may seem like a lot of work and may seem to take the surprise and expectation out of a week. You would expect to feel bound and shackled, but you will suddenly feel free to pursue your dreams.

Huge amounts of wasted time will vanish as you set up these automatic routines.

In order to build ritual into your life, start by taking an "audit" of your days to see what rituals you've already established, because whether we're aware of them or not, we all already have some established routines in our schedules. In fact, you might have some unhealthy rituals such as smoking or drinking, and you will want to limit or cut these from your life. "Show me where most of your rituals are and I'll show you what's important to you," Dr. Loehr says. When you do an "audit," write down what you do during every single waking hour — how do you carve up twenty-four hours? How do you carve up a week? Using the categories of rituals listed below, think about your day and try to see how many rituals you already have — do you have too few rituals? Do you have wrong, unhealthy rituals?

When you plan your day and your week, try to include as many rituals as possible from the categories listed below. Build rituals around what is important to you. For most people it is of utmost importance to create the best possible routines for the morning and the early part of the day. Dr. Loehr compares launching the day to launching a missile — if you launch the day badly, then your entire day will go badly. So pay attention to your morning routines — hygiene, reading the paper, preparing the children for school, walking the pets, and so on. Your morning routines should be so good that when you walk out of your house, you feel ready to tackle any problem you might encounter. Think about the rest of your day. If family time is important, then build rituals around that — this might mean spending time over dinner with your family, scheduling a spousal date for a Saturday night, or anything else you can think of. Locate the difficult moments of your day and build rituals around them. The rituals should become part of your life; and as stress increases, follow your routine more religiously in order to take control of your time and your life. Be sure to set up rituals for physical, emotional, and psychological health.

Sleep

No activity is more important to ritualize than sleep. Having a great routine that relaxes you and gets you to sleep and fixing a bedtime and a rising time will allow you to reap the maximum benefit from your biological clock. If you're having trouble sleeping, turn to the end of Part One, to the chapter titled "Maximize Alertness: Problem Solving," for a complete guideline on how to prepare for a restful night.

Meals

Foraging for food used to consume the human being's entire existence. Modern food-production techniques have freed a lot of time for us, yet many of us lose countless hours every week trying to choose what to eat, where to eat, and when to eat. By fixing mealtimes and planning in advance what to eat, you'll become vastly more efficient. This is not to steal away from dining as entertainment or part of socializing. Michael Crichton will pick one kind of lunch to eat every day during the months he's writing a novel. I've followed his example and will eat just one lunch for months on end. Since these meals are carefully designed to yield maximum mental energy, I get what I want out of the meal, even if the repetition becomes a little dull. You'll want to ingest performance-enhancing foods at strategic moments during the day.

Exercise

Since exercise has such powerful effect on brain energy and alertness, place your workouts at the times of day you most need them. For "evening people" or owls, a morning workout is a great way to boost alertness; for "morning people" or larks, an afternoon workout might provide just the right pick-me-up. While the activities may change, the time should not. If you choose to exercise mornings, use that time consistently.

Prime-time prep

In the morning, follow a two-step ritual that will help anchor you to the deepest, most important beliefs and desires in your life. First, make a "to do" list for the day. Second, spend ten minutes getting in touch with the things most important to you in life. You could turn on a music tape or you could do this exercise in silence. Think, visualize what you're about and what's important to you, and then connect the day's activities to that — connect today with the overall picture of what you're trying to accomplish in life. You might want to restructure your business, change the way you treat your employees, have more family time, have more time alone, or find time for spirituality. Dr. Loehr emphasizes that taking these ten minutes in the morning to contextualize the day in your life will help improve your follow-through.

Prime time

Being at your peak during the hours you should be at your best, what I call prime time, is the whole reason for ritual, whether you are a world-class pianist, sprinter, mother, or CEO. Prime time is the time to have maximum creativity and do your best work. Just as a surgeon has elaborate hand-washing techniques, or a pilot has set preflight routines, you should have rituals that relate to your job. Prep for prime time with excellent sleep, breakfast, and fitness rituals. Then set aside prime time as a ritual time to do your best work in a space specially set aside for prime time. Think of each day's prime time as being inviolable. Mark McCormack recognizes the benefit of prime time: "I am 110 percent a morning person and get my best work done very, very early in the morning." Morning is also prime time for superlawyer F. Lee Bailey: "My mental prime time is early in the morning, when others are sleeping and the phone is too."

Phone stacks

The telephone runs many people's lives. They feel they've worked a full day just because they answered all the calls. Keep a phone log for a week. Look at all the calls you really needed to take. Look at their timing. Create telephone time. Unless I have very important calls that require tremendous creative energy, which they usually don't, I save calling for the time of day when my creative energy is down and I don't feel I'm wasting time working the phones. Be brave enough to turn off your phone. Have a time of day when people can expect to get you, otherwise rely on voice mail. The rest of the world does. If someone really wants to reach you, they'll let you know.

Don't check voice mail hourly. Have a couple of key times when you check in. Don't let your phone time become your "prime" time.

I use a cell phone to return my calls at the end of the day during the ride home. By saving your calls till the end of the day, you carve out large amounts of creative time during the day. I'll also use rides to and from airports, time in airport lounges, and time waiting in lines to make calls. Calling during waiting or commuting time can be a pick-me-up and a great way to spend otherwise wasted time.

Dr. Loehr suggests ritualizing even the way you use the phone. For an important phone conversation, stand up while speaking and think of the conversation as a performance onstage. Your performance will improve and be more focused if you're standing tall; standing, your posture is probably better than when you're seated and hunched over. Use a headset to keep your hands free.

Digital stacks

Checking e-mail, Yahoo news, dinner menus, airline miles, stock prices, and myriad other places online can seem a predictably positive stack . . . but it can also become a highly addictive activity. Be wary of logging on too frequently, to the point that your e-mail runs your day. Have designated times to log on, then log off so you don't steal too much prime time from your day. By setting ritual times to log on, you can use the Web as a break or as a mood booster at the end of prime time.

Negative stacks

Take the things you really hate to do or things that put you in a bad mood and place them at times of the day when you have the greatest energy and resilience. There's no bigger mistake than approaching negative stacks when you are feeling weak and vulnerable. You'll be ineffective and look weak as well. Hold off making critical calls until you feel strong.

Planning tomorrow

In the waning hours of the day, take ten minutes to plan tomorrow. Make this a firm ritual so that you don't wander into the following day without a plan. Wandering into tomorrow without a plan is the most surefire way to kill prime time. I use a computer day planner to block out my activities so that there is clear structure to my day. Have one or two really key objectives; think about execution. Knowing that you have a plan of action for tomorrow's big problems will help you sleep better. If you think about it, most of us do schedule what we need to do the next day as we're falling asleep or, even worse, when we wake up in the wee hours. Those are two times when you will suffer the greatest anxieties about the problems ahead and have the fewest mental resources to deal with them. Just before you fall asleep or at 4:00 in the morning, problems will seem a lot blacker than they actually are. When you carve out an evening time to plan tomorrow, the day's pressure is off, so you'll have time to reflect and strategize about the coming day. Be sure to leave at least a half hour buffer for reading and relaxation before you turn in. Then when you rise in the morning, just put the plan into action so you lose the least amount of prime time.

Commuting

If you can't find time alone during the day and you commute by train or bus every day, use the commuting time to relax — switch off your cell phone, listen to music that relaxes you, read, use the commute for time alone. You could also use the commute for creative time. Bring your laptop and try writing. Regardless of traffic or weather delays, you'll feel a sense of accomplishment.

Travel

If you're a frequent traveler, take the time to ritualize your departure. Don't make it a fresh adventure each time out the door. Leave a much bigger buffer than you need to make a plane, car, or bus. If you're not going to use the travel time as time alone, bring with you work to do: phone calls to make, papers to read, messages to write. Have a positive stack of these activities so you actually look forward to the time you'll have to spend. I return phone calls on the way to the airport, bring along journal articles to read, and look forward to browsing for magazines at the newsstand. I also always leave a buffer of at least one flight after my departure in case my original flight is canceled. Equally important is that I always check the weather forecast for the departure and arrival cities as well as for any connecting cities. Know when your plane just isn't going to get there. The other day I had a flight from La Guardia through Chicago's O'Hare to San Diego. I checked the weather forecast, found Chicago was down to minimums, with fog and low visibility, then considered the next connecting city, San Francisco, and ultimately made my way through Los Angeles. Neither of the other flights made it on time. If you're playing the upgrade game, try to have it sorted out before you arrive at the airport so that you're not frantically waiting until the last minute to find out that you have a middle seat in steerage surrounded by recently released burglars on their way to a halfway house. If you fly a lot, set flight routines, which might include getting up and walking during the flight, not drinking caffeine, bringing along pleasurable reading, or bringing along blinders to block out light and let you sleep.

Stress breaks

If you know certain meetings or professional activities stress you out, plan a stress break. I do that late each afternoon, with a half hour of weight training at the gym. Dr. Loehr suggests that during the work day, you take fifteen- to twenty-minute "recovery breaks" every hour and a half. You can hydrate, walk, or deep-breathe during your break. The break is a little episode of recovery to detoxify, rejuvenate, and experience a rebirth that will allow you to return to work more focused.

Play time

You'll be dull and less productive without it, so schedule play time. Really go for it, so your ordinary concerns fade deeply into the background. Whether you're watching plays, operas, or movies, or playing tennis or soccer with kids, or building model airplanes, make sure to play!

The chapter "Plan the Biologically Successful Day" sets up a series of sample rituals to help you design your own biologically successful day. Remember, wherever you have a problem area, building lots of rituals around the difficulty will help you stay in control of the situation.

Step 9: Preserve Mental Capital

―――― ⁞⁞⁞⁞⁞⁞ ――――

We have a flawed notion that the most successful authors, poets, painters, executives, doctors, researchers, moms and dads, all have unending mental energy. Would that it were true! The fact is that we all have a certain quantity of mental capital to spend in a given day. To be truly great, we have to be just as careful about preserving mental capital as about creating it. This chapter outlines the worst destroyers of mental capital. In America today, tense energy is what we see the most of, as characterized by Kramer's hyperantics in the sitcom *Seinfeld*. We are a nation full of individuals paralyzed by anxiety and tension. Pathologically high tension levels kill mental energy and with it productivity, across the board. Only by stripping away tension are we able to gain the greatest measure of unfettered mental energy. You may find that you are a very positive person, but that you are still robbed of many creative hours each day by excessive tension and stress because you can't concentrate long enough to get your quality work done. Or, if you often have a negative mood or are frankly depressed, you may find that anxiety further robs you of a happy, productive life.

> **CONVENTIONAL WISDOM:** Get up a buzz —
> energy at any cost.
> **THE BIOLOGY OF SUCCESS:** Calm energy is the
> ideal mood for superior mental performance.

The Biology of Calm

In studies of students, calm energy predicts best who can study the most effectively. Robert E. Thayer, Ph.D., in *The Origin of Everyday Moods,* describes four categories of mood: calm energy, calm tiredness, tense energy, and tense tiredness. Feelings about energy and tiredness indicate readiness for action or need for recuperation or rest. Feelings about tension or calmness are signals about how safe or threatened we feel.

Take the brief self-test below to assess your degree of anxiety. Once again, Robert L. Spitzer, M.D., Chief of Biometric Research at the New York State Psychiatric Institute, has kindly provided the test.

Self-Test

For each, please answer with one of the following options:

A. NOT AT ALL
B. SEVERAL DAYS
C. MORE THAN HALF THE DAYS
D. NEARLY EVERY DAY

Over the last 4 weeks, how often have you been bothered by:

_____ 1. Feeling nervous, anxious, on edge, or worrying a lot about different things?

_____ 2. Feeling restless so that it is hard to sit still?

_____ 3. Getting tired very easily?

_____ 4. Muscle tension, aches, or soreness?

_____ 5. Trouble falling asleep or staying asleep?

_____ 6. Trouble concentrating on things, such as reading a book or watching TV?

_____ 7. Becoming easily annoyed or irritable?

Diagnosis

• If you answered MORE THAN HALF THE DAYS or NEARLY EVERY DAY to question 1 and answered MORE THAN HALF THE DAYS or NEARLY EVERY DAY for three or more of questions 2–7 you may suffer from a real anxiety disorder. You may want to consider medication and psychotherapy, which you will have to discuss with a physician.

You'll want to consider supplementing that treatment with the measures described below.

- If you answered SEVERAL DAYS to three or more questions, you have in your life substantial tension that is seriously impeding your ability to attain a positive mood and maintain mental energy. You'll also want to consider many of the measures listed below.

How to Cut Anxiety and Improve Energy

Many of the Steps in Part One, for example music therapy or creating quiet space, can help cut anxiety, but the most effective single means of cutting tension is exercise, which also builds physical energy. If exercise turns you off, you may be surprised to learn that very little is needed to cut tension — five minutes can take a stiff bite out of whatever tension you are feeling. Tai chi, Qigong, and deep-breathing exercises all cut tension and are easy to practice in the office. Qigong is an ancient Chinese medicinal art, similar to tai chi, which can work wonders for tension. Special diets also cut tension by removing the foods that make you anxious and adding the foods that create calm.

Dealing with Anxiety

Now, not all anxiety is a bad thing. We know that some anxiety is critical for survival. If our prehistoric ancestors hadn't worried about being eaten by a predator, they would have failed to take preventive measures. We should allow our brain the opportunity to scan the horizon for trouble spots and take action, but not when we are the least energized and most anxious, because we'll be least creative about finding a solution then. Imagine waking at 3:00 A.M. in an anxious state. You have no energy resources or creative power to find a solution; you're just left with anxiety-provoking problems. You mull them over as your heart rate begins to climb. Pretty soon you're tossing and turning . . . many hours before you can get up and take action. This endless worry that we aim at problems rarely solves them and simply saps energy. It's unhealthy, too. The journal

Circulation, published by the American Heart Association, reports that worry increases the risk of heart attack.

Paradoxically, people who endlessly worry don't often come up with good solutions. They would be far better off concentrating on building a positive mood with less anxiety. In that state they can far more easily take on their problems and those of the world. Better to face big problems in the morning, when your energy level is highest and tension is lowest.

What Destroys Mental Energy

Tension, anxiety, and a foul mood can also be created by how we run our day. Subconsciously, we try to modify our moods throughout the day with sugary or fatty foods and stimulating drugs. Many of these, however, are mood wreckers. While certain foods and drugs may give you an immediate boost, research shows us that the boost is temporary and followed by a marked and prolonged lower mood. A better strategy is to recognize the change in mood and treat it with any of the measures in the preceding chapters.

Any of the following drugs, nutrients, synthetic substances, activities, or psychological states can disturb your natural biological rhythms, sleep-wake cycles, or even neurotransmitter levels. As important as building mental energy is, preserving that mental capital is even more important. Below is a list of what to avoid.

"XXX"-rated mood wreckers

POOR SLEEP, OR DISTURBED SLEEP-WAKE CYCLES
Getting a poor night's sleep is the best way to ruin your mental capital for the next twenty-four hours. Whether from too much alcohol, caffeine, emotional turmoil, food, or activity late into the evening, sleep disturbance will exhaust you and leave you looking older and more haggard. The problem solving chapter at the end of Part One has many helpful suggestions for improving your sleep.

ANGER
Anger causes the most rapid and profound of all mood changes. The surge in adrenaline, the stress hormone cortisol, and other hor-

mones will get your heart rate and blood pressure up and keep it up. Since resurrecting a good mood after a bout of real anger may also take hours, anger can wreck your whole day. When you get angry, the major victim is yourself.

PERFECTIONIST ATTITUDE

Many successful people are not perfectionists. In fact striving for perfection can be exactly the *wrong* goal. Here's why: When you're a perfectionist, you are basically telling yourself, "I'm working on something that I don't think I can do." When you define your work in such a perfectionistic way, you create a self-defeating, disheartening situation in which you're literally working on things you don't think you can accomplish. In fact, people who are depressed or in a bad mood tend to adopt a perfectionistic style. They set standards or goals for themselves that exceed what they have time to do or are actually capable of doing. Always thinking as a perfectionist prolongs your state of feeling bad because you can never achieve what you set out to do.

THE WRONG CROWD

The people around us dramatically affect how we feel about ourselves. A high-energy crowd at a parade lifts your mood, while hanging with a bunch of grouches complaining about work is sure to drop it. People form a neural network around us, connecting us to each other emotionally like one nerve cell to another. The chapter "Practice Emotional Broadcasting" in Part Two has much more on interaction with people.

NEGATIVE STACKING

We all have unpleasant duties — say, the phone call we hate to make. One reason we hate to make it is simple anxiety, the other is that it makes us feel bad. I'm a big believer in launching those bad calls at a time when you are most resilient. That can be in the morning when your mood is rising or just after exercise when you feel bulletproof. I like to insulate myself by tackling distasteful activities and then backing myself up with a series of positive activities. Stacking too long a list of negative duties at the wrong time of day will certainly drag you down! When you do tackle activities you dislike, anticipate the stress and use it to your advantage so that you are more powerful and effective. The Step "Set a Ritual" provides a thorough guideline on how to avoid negative stacking.

ASPARTAME

Critics link aspartame to afternoon depression, anxiety, and truly foul moods. You'll find it in diet colas and other diet foods. Industry advocates and the FDA, however, see no major problems with aspartame. There is a veritable internet war between pro and anti aspartame factions. See how you believe aspartame affects you and decide for yourself.

CAFFEINE

Caffeine gives you a great short-term boost, usually for an hour after you ingest the soft drink, tea, or coffee. Although you could try to pump yourself with caffeine all day long, the effect is lessened with each new dose, and at the end of the day you'll be tired and anxious. When you try to fall asleep, you'll find yourself staring at the ceiling. I'll admit to having been a caffeine, aspartame addict. The first hit of Diet Coke in the morning made me feel just terrific. I'd hit myself again and again, with less and less result. Finally, in the late afternoon, I'd turned into a real monster: grumpy, anxious, and mildly depressed. Unfortunately, this came right at the time when I had to be at my best, because evening news would be on television. When I gave up Diet Coke (I still drink the real thing on occasion), my energy surged and the tension evaporated. I found I could sit and work for far longer periods of time. Best of all, I began having the most refreshing sleep in years. Remember that craving caffeine is usually a symptom of too little sleep or poor-quality sleep. If you have to have caffeine, try it at midmorning after a big, hearty breakfast. That way you won't suffer the double blow of a rapidly falling blood sugar and an attendant adrenaline release. The dropping blood sugar and rising adrenaline are sure to leave you shaky and in a poor mood.

ALCOHOL

Alcohol has an almost instant energizing effect, largely through the relief of tension that it delivers. Unfortunately, that tension rises again in about ninety minutes and is accompanied by a substantial loss of energy and drop in mood. However, the worst effect of alcohol on mood is its effect on the quality of your sleep, what the experts call your sleep architecture. A few drinks at night will ruin the quality of your sleep and decrease your performance the following day. Even moderate drinking causes a decline in productivity at work.

FOODS

Many of us use foods as the drugs that keep us going during the day. We often don't realize that foods can cause a sharp deterioration in mental energy and mood. Here's how:

- Big meals: Big meals really do kill a good mood. They steal away blood supply from the rest of the body and leave you sluggish and sleepy.

- Fatty meals: Fatty foods take a major draw on mental energy. They feel great going down, but a large fatty meal can also quickly drag down your mood and mental energy.

- Sugary foods: These foods, from donuts and coffee rolls to candy bars, do boost your mood . . . again, for less than an hour. That's how long it takes for your blood sugar to rise and plummet. You could eat these foods all day long to keep your mood up but you'll find yourself stressed at day's end and packing on a considerable amount of fat. The foods you want to avoid are characterized by a high glycemic index, meaning that they will cause large increases in your blood sugar level (see the table on pages 215–216). These foods present their greatest danger to you when they are eaten alone as a snack without any other foods to buffer them. Larry Christensen and his colleagues from Texas A&M reported that diets from which sugar has been eliminated led to decreases in depression.

These are just quick points on how to prevent foods from wrecking your mood. Step 4, "Eat for Mental Energy," should have already given you a detailed plan of how to use foods to maximize your mental capital.

Mental Capital

Great writers may start writing at 5:00 A.M. but be out of fresh ideas by 9:00 A.M. Top executives may have extremely strong mornings and fade in the afternoon. The key is to spend that mental capital wisely. Imagine having a great novelist wasting precious mental capital going over old phone bills in her prime morning writing hours, when so much more time is available later in the day when her most valuable mental capital has already been spent. The following chapter, "Plan the Biologically Successful Day," will help you plan how to spend your mental capital wisely.

Plan the Biologically
Successful Day

———— |||||| ————

A doctor comes into her office at 7:00 A.M. to catch up on paperwork. She's already had two cups of coffee and is racing against the clock before starting rounds at the hospital. By the end of the day she's seen thirty patients. A manager sloshes down an Egg McMuffin while running down the ramp to an aircraft. After a daylong stopover at a plant, he's figured out how to restructure its operation. A top money manager sells a billion-dollar fund during a road show. A violinist completes her audition for the Boston Symphony Orchestra. Each one of these people functions well and accomplishes great feats. But by nightfall, what kind of day have they had? The doctor is too exhausted to play with her children. The plant manager has to wade through several cocktails before he can even begin to think about heading home. The top financial manager is too tired for a workout, and the violinist doesn't have the energy to practice any further. Each one of these people may have had a day full of accomplishments, but from a biological vantage point, it was a disaster. Their brains and bodies functioned, but at certain times during the day only at a crawl. The biologically successful day is far different. You enter with eager enthusiasm and strength which builds throughout the morning. Your afternoon is engineered to deal with flagging midday biological rhythms. By evening you are refreshed and ready for family, a social evening, reading, or writing. My late friend George Sheehan always said the golden rule of life was first to be a good animal. That means having a day that feels great, having an entire day during which you are biologically at your peak. The key principle of the biologically successful day is understanding how much your body and brain chemistry change over the course of the day. What you are in the morning is entirely different from what you are in the afternoon and evening. Scheduling the perfect day accounts for knowing how your body functions during each period of the day and how you can best enhance that performance.

CONVENTIONAL WISDOM: "Have a great day."
THE BIOLOGY OF SUCCESS: Make it a great day.

Many of us believe we can't have it all. However, with careful structure and rituals, you can have a biologically and professionally successful day every day. The biologically successful day utilizes everything you've learned so far in this book, combining a firm understanding of your own biological clock with the ritual of activities that optimize every part of your day. Imagine rising in the morning completely rested, coasting through the day with energy to spare, and cruising into the evening still brimming with energy. The unique high concept here is strategically placing rituals and stacks of activities to get the maximum benefit out of your biological clock.

The Biology of a Biologically Successful Day

The biologically successful day enhances all of your natural biological rhythms so that both the valleys and peaks provide a higher level of mental energy and the most time at peak brain power.

You'll find in this chapter a concrete sample daily plan for managing your moods and building positive mental energy. Remember, the single most important part of manipulating your daily mood is matching your activities to fit these biological rhythms. It is pretty straightforward: Synchronize your most creative time with your most creative activities. Synchronize your low-energy time with reading and planning. It may seem a strange way to run your day, always chasing down activities that make us feel good, but that's what many of us already do unconsciously. The trouble is that we chase down activities that are harmful to mood — alcohol, sugar binges, caffeine, hours of watching TV.

Guarding prime time

Consider your prime time your long-term business priorities time and your off-peak time your busywork time. Sure, the busywork has to be done, but not at the expense of accomplishing your long-term career goals. So if you have a big report to author, a computer program to write, a Web page to design, a conference to construct, be sure the decks are clear. The most important part of planning your day is realizing when you are capable of producing the best results. For "larks," morning is a time of high energy and low tension, when you can focus, create, write. Afternoon for most people is a tough time, since energy levels sink as tension begins to rise. For "owls," the evening may be the best time to work, study, or write. The key is to design your day by building a fortress around the time when you know you are most productive and weeding out all peripheral activities. You'll feel much better once you've got a good chunk of highly creative time behind you. The reason that time-management programs often fail is that you're not dealing with a fully charged battery all day long. You need as best you can to schedule your most creative and energetic activities for when your brain is best suited to tackle them. For instance, Vladimir Horowitz used to give concerts, by preference, only at 4:00 P.M. on Sunday afternoons! William F. Buckley also prefers afternoons: "Late afternoon is best for me."

Adapting to off-peak

Friends, competitors, and colleagues may give you the impression that they are "on" at all times, that their mood never wavers from flagrant mania, yet every emotion throughout the day does not have to approach euphoria; in fact, it can't. But that doesn't mean that the varying emotions and moods can't be very productive. Find activities — such as reading, planning, making phone calls, cleaning up your desk, going over your finances — that take less creative energy and better suit your low-energy state.

The Biologically Successful Day

Below is an ideal daily schedule based purely on optimal biological function. If you're a real "lark," you could shift this an hour or so earlier.

Morning prime

6:30 A.M.

- Use full-intensity light: Rely on natural sunlight in the summer and the artificial light of a dawn simulator in the winter. Light strongly reinforces the setting of the biological clock and helps bring most rhythms that follow during the day to a high degree of regularity. Administering light early in the morning is the single most important thing you do to synchronize your alertness pacemaker. Using artificial light, you can choose to rise at any time, even 3:00 A.M. Just make certain it's the same time every day.

7 A.M. RISING

Up and at 'em! The most rigid part of your daily schedule should be a fixed time to wake up and get up! Hormone levels are still at a natural low, so here's how to enhance your morning.

- Drink a pure protein beverage just after rising. I make a soy protein shake as soon as I'm out of bed.

- Build an artificial first peak to your day with exercise to oxygenate the brain. I do an hour on the stair machine, building intensity through the hour and spiking it with fifteen one-minute intervals. If your workout is weak, add a "motivator" to get your blood sugar on the rise. I add a "motivator" to my morning protein drink — soy protein powder with a scoop or two of Twin Lab's Optifuel II, a banana, and ice. Sounds like a lot of calories, but you'll burn twice as many. Play motivational music. It's corny, but I'll turn on *The Sound of Music* or the Rachmaninoff Piano Concerto Number 3 as a boost to get up and get going.

- After your workout, continue having breakfast. I like to eat cantaloupe and uncooked oatmeal with yogurt. In its raw state, oatmeal causes an even smaller rise in your blood sugar and gives you even more staying power.

- Socialize: Dr. Michael Smolensky of the University of Texas School of Public Health has shown that in order to jump-start mood, most of us need socialization in the early morning, and yet this is precisely when many of us aren't motivated physically or emotionally to interact with others. This isolation and lack of motivation can set the tone for the day. So on your way to work and for the first few minutes at the office, take a little time to socialize before sitting down for morning prime time. My wife builds mental energy in the morning by making a quick round of phone calls to buoy her spirits before settling down to work.

8:00 A.M.–1:00 P.M.: PRIME TIME

- Take advantage of the body's rapidly rising energy level and low level of tension. Don't waste it! Use this time for key presentations, speeches, writing, creative meetings, surgery, painting, practicing a musical instrument, or any other activity that is promoting your life career goal. Great artists, writers, and thinkers often use the early morning to do their best work. In the crazy world we live in today, the early morning is also a time before the phone rings, before the fax machines start spitting out data, before the market opens, in short, before we are driven by other people's needs rather than our own.

- Take caffeine without sugar if you need a mental breakthrough at midmorning. It's the last time during the day that you should use caffeine. Once your pacemaker is fully synced, you probably won't need it.

- Avoid all sugary and starchy snacks.

- Play energetic and inspiring music.

- Extend your morning peak as long as possible before eating lunch. That's why a big breakfast is so important for making it all last.

Off-peak

Now larks are beginning to fade while owls may still be coming on strong. However, both will suffer a sizable drop in mood and mental energy during the afternoon.

1:30 P.M. LUNCH

- High protein to start — for example chicken or fish.

- Eat small to moderate amounts of high-fiber carbohydrates and very low-glycemic-index foods. Beans are best to keep you satisfied throughout the day.

2:00 P.M.–3:30 P.M.

Use this time to follow through on morning initiatives.

3:30 P.M.–5:00 p.m.

This is the dull zone. Take the floor of this valley and raise it.

- Take a fifteen-minute nap. Unlike snack foods, a brief fifteen-minute nap will make you feel great without packing on the pounds. Once you've trained yourself to nap, you'll feel far sharper and more energetic after a nap than after a snack.

- Take a ten-minute walk or exercise break to revive yourself.

- Stack positive activities, including reinforcing phone calls.

- Use the downturn in mood to read or research quietly. The key is to be certain to keep tension low as well. Playing soothing classical music is a good way to get into the groove.

- Don't eat junk foods: Recapture your mental strength with activity and napping. Don't eat to recover!

- Don't pull out your major strategic plan or high-powered to-do list and start executing it. You'll wonder how you ever had the strength to make it up. It will be discouraging and frustrating. Remember to execute in the same mood in which you created the plan. So if you were highly charged one morning and figured out a killer strategy, don't start working the phones and recruiting converts when your mood is low.

5:00 P.M.–7:00 p.m.: REGENERATE STRENGTH

- Daytime energy dips to its lowest point in the late afternoon, around five o'clock, something employers have long understood.

This is the best time to use activity to reinvigorate yourself. 5:00–7:00 P.M. is when most health clubs hit their peak. Although you may be mentally fatigued, it's when your body may be at its performance peak. See if you don't run a minute per mile faster or cycle three miles an hour faster or stair-step two gradients higher at 5:00 P.M. than at 7:00 A.M.

Early evening

7:00 P.M.–8:30 p.m.

- Eat a very small dinner for peak performance. I have a Boca burger and a sweet potato — that's got lots of bulk and fiber without many calories. It's lean enough to give me a very strong evening.

- Good conversation builds positive emotional ties. This is the best family time and social time. Use it to build motivation and energy for evening prime.

Evening prime

Many of the world's great battle plans and political campaigns were created during this time and on into the wee hours, when distractions are at a minimum and calm sets in. The brain energy kicks in again to give you a second prime time. Without the phones, visitors, and other interruptions, it's also a period of surprising calm.

8:30 P.M.–10:30 P.M.
Write or read.

10:30 P.M.–11 P.M.
Plan your to-do list for the following day. Listen to calming music.

11:00 P.M.–11:30 P.M.
Set a regular bedtime. Practice your sleep hygiene routine. That means beginning prep at 11:00 P.M. Have some great reading material left. Be ready to fall asleep at 11:30 P.M. if you need a full seven and a half to eight hours.

That's the basic sample blueprint. You'll want to custom design your own day based on your own schedule, job requirements, strengths, and weaknesses. If you're a strong lark, you may find your evening prime is not as strong as you wish. If you're a strong owl, you may have trouble with early morning prime. In either case, a strong set of rituals implementing the measures in Part One of this book will place you squarely on the road to success. One last point to remember. Most of us fool ourselves when waging the actual number of productive hours we have per day. Better to have three very strong creative hours than to spend twelve hours struggling to work. Once you've earned your keep, take the time to play hard and invigorate yourself.

Maximize Alertness:
Problem Solving

———— |||||| ————

Before the advent of electricity and jet aircraft, there was no jet lag, shift work, or time sickness. But those days are in the remote past. When we disrupt our natural rhythms, we are setting our biological clocks to the wrong time. Let's take a look at the problems caused by disrupting the natural rhythms set by our biological clocks and how to fix them.

Problem #1:
Monday-Morning Jet Lag

One of the major indications that the biological clock is not doing its job right is malaise of the sort you feel after an all-nighter. In addition to feeling sleepy, you experience an affective, emotional discomfort. You feel grouchy and tense. Many of us have the misfortune of living on a 24-hour planet with a biological clock that times out a 24.5-hour day. This means that when it is time for bed at the end of a regular day, many of us still have an extra hour of wakefulness, which means that our clock really shifts patterns of sleep and wakefulness "westward" by about half an hour a day — so, you may wake up in New York, but by late evening, your biological clock is in Chicago. If you actually do stay up later, you risk getting up an hour later in the morning; and the delayed exposure to light in the morning will shift your biological clock even later, throwing your pacemaker out of kilter. That's precisely what causes Monday-morning jet lag. When you go to bed much later on the weekend, which many of us do, your clock is going to be pushed westward. So if on Friday and Saturday you've gone to bed at 3:00 A.M. instead of 10:00 P.M., then slept in until 10:00 or 11:00 A.M. on Saturday and Sunday, here's what happens: when you rise on Monday morning, your clock is in Hawaii, but your body is in New York! That is, your body thinks it's 2:00 A.M. Eastern time, when your alarm goes off at 7:00 A.M. Ouch . . . it's Monday-morning jet lag!

Solutions

Every top expert says rule number one for maintaining your biological clock is rising at the exact same time every morning. Every extra hour you sleep in resets your time clock by an hour. Recovering will take you one day for every hour you sleep in. That means that "sleeping in" on Saturdays and Sundays can put you out of whack until midweek. You should obviously try to get to bed at the same time each evening. If you can't, still be certain to get up at the same time, even if you've been out until 3:00 A.M. Get up, do some exercise, have breakfast . . . then when you hit the post-lunch dip described below, take a nap. You'd be surprised that after a big night out, you'll actually feel worse if you sleep in late, say until 11:00 A.M., than if you get up and suffer the consequences.

Problem #2: The Graveyard Shift

Twenty percent of the U.S. population has to rotate their work shift on a regular basis — say the 8:00 A.M. to 4:00 P.M., then the 4:00 P.M. to midnight, then the midnight to 8:00 A.M. Working day and night, shift workers constantly have to reorient their sleep/wake cycle. Some individuals are simply unable to adapt their cycles and leave work within six months; then there are those who can do shift work for twenty-five to thirty years! Data is primarily on men, as they are dominant in that 20 percent. Individuals who tolerate shift work have a biological time structure that is quite flexible; their peak-to-trough variations of the specific rhythms important for shift work are at relatively low amplitude — so they shift very easily. For these people, very low energy is channeled into the circadian cycle, so that when they shift they can do so relatively rapidly. But even for these well-adapted souls, there is a cost. Around the age of forty-five to fifty something now called the "Shift Work Male Adaptation

Syndrome" appears. This disease occurs when workers are on the night rotation, and is marked by a persistent inability to sleep during the day. Workers start taking sleep aids, drugs, and alcohol, but nothing completely solves the problem. The individual becomes sleep deprived while on the night shift; his mood is low, his risk of accidents rises, self-esteem and confidence plummet, and performance drops. He also starts to pack on the pounds. The social consequences are frightening: emotional intolerance in work, marriage, and family life. Dr. Allan Geliebter of the Obesity Research Center at St. Luke's–Roosevelt Hospital Center in New York reported that during his study, hospital late-shift workers gained an average of 9.5 pounds, while day workers gained only about 2 pounds. Worse still, researchers find that shift workers' blood pressure does not dip at night as it should, which increases the risk of heart disease. Research also indicates that in order to correct permanently all these ills, patients must give up the shift cycle and become consistent in their sleep-wake cycle. After years of working in shifts, reorientation to standard habits typically takes from six months to a year. Because of the prevalence of the "Shift Work Male Adaptation Syndrome," companies are now making it a priority to set a more biologically adaptable shift system and teach the worker about his biology, and even more importantly, about his chronobiology.

Eve Van Cauter, Ph.D., Research Professor in Medicine at the University of Chicago, says, "We humans are unique in our capacity to ignore circadian signals and to maintain wakefulness despite an increased pressure to go to sleep." Unlike most animals who steal sleep at various intervals throughout the twenty-four-hour period, the human being sleeps in consolidated shifts and can to a certain degree willfully change these shifts. And yet, the more we ignore our circadian rhythm, the more difficult it becomes to ignore it. The longer we ignore our need, the greater the desire to satiate that need — this is the premise underlying our homeostatic forces. And the homeostatic drive that keeps processes balanced in the body kicks in with sleep deprivation as it does with hunger. The more we starve ourselves of food, the more food we need to eat to recover;

and, similarly, the longer we go without sleep, the more urgently our homeostatic forces will tell us that we're sleepy, the more tired we become, and the greater our need for sleep.

Solutions

Pick one shift and stick with it. On weekends, don't go back to another schedule; wake at the same time during the weekend as you would during the week. Be extraordinarily careful when changing from one shift to another. Your biggest risks during the switchover are driving to and from work and safety on the job. Taking melatonin does not appear to help workers on rotating shifts adjust to working nights, report researchers at Vanderbilt University.

Problem #3: Daily Mood Swings

Most of us wake up in the lowest energy state of the day. That low energy level gradually rises to a peak between 11:00 A.M. and early afternoon. By late afternoon, we have our lowest mental energy level since waking and our highest level of tension — this is the most unproductive time of day. We then experience a smaller energy peak in the early evening. You want to be aware of these mood and energy swings so you can either plan your day around them or find ways to make them more productive.

Here are the two key troughs most of us hit every day.

Morning blahs

It is perfectly natural to feel down first thing in the morning, because from the perspective of your biological clock everything is down. Sometimes this feeling can last all morning, but don't mistakenly think that your early morning low will necessarily last all day long. Don't be deceived by the attitudes of the cheerful actors in the cornflakes ad we talked about in Step 1, "Activate the Alertness Triggers"; it's probably not the first thing in the morning when they are putting on those radiant smiles for the camera. Chances are they produced the ad midmorning, and by then you too will be smiling! Remind yourself that an hour from now you will be feeling much better.

Solutions

A great breakfast gets your blood sugar climbing fast.

Exercise in the morning increases brain oxygenation and gets all your hormones humming far earlier than your biological clock would. And a good night's rest will help you awaken refreshed.

Great sleep preparation, described below, will get you the night's sleep you need to wake up fresh and relaxed.

- Avoid caffeine. Coffee, tea, and even chocolate will keep you awake for several hours after you ingest them. Taken in the evening, they can destroy most of an otherwise good night's sleep. Many Americans are so sensitive that even a Diet Coke in the early afternoon can wreck a good night's sleep.

- Avoid nicotine, which is a stronger stimulant than caffeine. If you're smoking or using nicotine patches or inhalers, try to quit early in the day.

- Avoid alcohol before bedtime. Alcohol disturbs both REM (active, dreaming) and NREM (deep, restorative) sleep, and you will awaken not feeling rested. Even a single drink from the early evening on can destroy sleep architecture . . . and degrade your productivity at work.

- Eat a healthy, balanced diet — don't go to bed hungry or uncomfortably full, because either state can make it difficult to fall asleep or stay asleep. If you're hungry, have a light snack at least half an hour before lying down to sleep.

- Exercise regularly, but not a few hours before bedtime, since physical exertion then will awaken you. The only exception is sexual orgasm — satisfying sex that is free of anxiety will for most people help induce restful sleep.

- Create a peaceful, comfortable bedroom environment:
  - Make sure your mattress is not too hard or too soft.
  - Regulate the air temperature so that it's not too hot or too cold and the humidity so that it's not too dry or too humid.
  - If your room overlooks a noisy street, use earplugs or a low-sound-generating machine such as an air conditioner to drown out noise.

— Make sure you have enough shades to prevent the very early morning light from waking you.

— Keep your room and your bedsheets and pillows clean.

— Don't let pets lie on your bed while you sleep.

• Associate your room with rest rather than work or quarrel.

• Create and maintain a bedtime ritual. For example, spend a few minutes reading for pleasure every night.

• Take a warm bath before bedtime.

• Try relaxation techniques such as meditation or slow deep breathing before sleeping. I've learned Qigong, which is a wonderful combination of meditation, rhythmic arm movements, and extraordinarily long and deep breathing. To learn it properly you'll need a Qigong instructor, now available in most metropolitan areas and easily found in the yellow pages.

Keep a sleep log to document your daily sleeping/waking habits and identify problems that are causing you sleepless nights.

Research shows that many of us may ideally need ten hours of sleep a day for optimal performance. With our busy schedules, we're lucky if we get eight. Be sure not to get less than eight hours if you don't want your mood and performance to deteriorate. When you are sleeping eight hours a night and keeping a regular schedule, the interaction of the circadian and homeostatic processes will help you to maintain a high, stable level of performance. You will find yourself working more quickly, more efficiently, and more successfully. So schedule eight hours of sleep a night. Mark them in your calendar. Good night, sleep tight, and don't let your sleep debt rise.

The post-lunch dip

The post-lunch dip is a period of decreased alertness which strikes between 1:00 P.M. and 4:00 P.M. During these hours, work performance suffers, people in dimly lit rooms are apt to nod off, and if you're on the road, the likelihood of having a car accident increases. Studies suggest that as many as 50 percent of fatal highway accidents are caused by drivers falling asleep or briefly nodding off behind the wheel . . . and the most frequent times of accidents are, unsurprisingly, 4:00 A.M. and 4:00 P.M.!

The body clock provides the scientific reason behind the post-lunch dip. Daily fluctuations in body temperature, hormone levels, and other physiological cycles place us at a low ebb in the afternoon, in contrast to the high ebbs of peak alertness in the morning when we are sleep satiated and in the early evening when our pacemaker is at its peak. By late afternoon we have our lowest mental energy since waking, our highest level of tension, and, as a result, our least productive time of day.

After lunch, as your blood redirects to the stomach and digestive system and away from your other vital organs, your mood falls to a low point. Do you crave sugar or other carbos mid to late afternoon? When your energy is sinking to its lowest while your tension is climbing to its daily high, carbos feel good because they help make brain serotonin to cut anxiety and tension. Just as important, carbos raise blood sugar levels, which is key, because in the afternoon your insulin levels will peak while your glucose is at a minimum and as a result your body does not have as much sugar to metabolize for energy. Furthermore, because of all the activities and exercise of the day, lactic acid is building up in your muscles, and that makes you feel tired. All of these factors result in the late-afternoon slump that chronobiologists have named the "post-lunch dip."

How bad is your post-lunch dip? According to Ralph Morris, Ph.D., Professor of Pharmacology at the University of Illinois, how quickly you recover from that post-lunch dip depends on whether you are a lark or an owl as well as on your environment (what you do in the afternoon, whether you sleep, go to a happy hour, are bored, excited, etc.). After the post-lunch dip, without proper intervention, the lark who has been up since the early-morning hours may stay down emotionally, possibly physically, for the rest of the day. Since owls are used to getting a sluggish start, they will pick up better after lunch — the low point of the day makes less of an impression on them; they always feel better in the afternoon!

Solutions

Different societies have come up with different ways to manage this slump. The English invented "teatime" as a solution: lots of caffeine and cakes to prop up their flagging energies. The Spanish adopted the afternoon siesta, while the Americans simply threw in the towel and declared five o'clock quitting time. Unfortunately, the early quitting-time strategy robs us of one of the most productive times of day, the early evening. The most effective solutions are as follows:

- Have a light high-protein lunch. That builds alertness neurotransmitters, described in Step 4, which fight the tendency toward lethargy. Ironically, the post-lunch dip is misnamed — it occurs even without a meal, but a big carbohydrate lunch exacerbates the situation and makes you even more tired.

- Plan a lunchtime exercise break to raise artificially all your important hormonal levels in order to create an afternoon peak. If you don't have time to exercise, take a quick walk outside.

- Schedule less taxing activities for the post-lunch dip. If possible, you should do most of your mentally demanding work in the morning or early evening rather than trudging unproductively during the post-lunch dip.

- Plan a midafternoon high-quality snack to fight the late-afternoon rise in tension. Also, consider drinking tea or an ice-cold juice.

- Take a power nap. If you're sleep-deprived, take a 15- to 30-minute power nap. More than 30 minutes will make you groggy. Churchill did it; Ben Franklin did it. Power naps will immediately improve your productivity. Remember that napping is the low-calorie alternative to using food to improve mental energy. It's also far more effective and less likely to backfire. My father has always been a big believer in napping. Other than exercising, there is no better way to immediately offset a foul mood. If you're anxious or stressed to the limit, you probably won't be able to nap, and exercise is still a better strategy. However, if you're jet-lagged, sleep-deprived, and feeling low on energy, far better than turning to food is to take a good 20-minute nap.

- Monitor your mood. Most of us have no conscious idea of what kind of mood we are in unless we're on top of the world or down in the sewer. Keep in mind that although mental energy is not synonymous with a positive mood, a positive mood is the most effective means of creating mental energy. Only by monitoring your mood during a given day will you know when you need a boost and when you are already in a positive, creative mood.

Problem #4: Pacemaker Mood Illness

In day-to-day life your biological clock influences mood changes, but ultimately changes in mood reflect the synchrony between your lifestyle and your pacemaker. In other words, if you are very regular about when you wake up and when you go to bed and you are on a day schedule, then your pacemaker is going to adjust itself in harmony with your lifestyle and you are going to achieve a good relationship between your lifestyle and your clock — you will have stable levels of mood. However, if you are very irregular in your sleep pattern, in when you go to bed and wake up, you might induce not just a mood swing but an actual mood illness.

New research shows that disruptions in sleep routines trigger mania in people with manic-depression, a disorder characterized by violent mood swings alternating from severe depression to mania. Ellen Frank, M.D., of the University of Pittsburgh Medical Center's Western Psychiatric Institute and Clinic, reports: "We need to help people with manic-depressive disorder develop sound routines in order to protect their biological clock from disturbances." By normalizing their sleep patterns, patients with manic-depressive illnesses may add to the protective effect of mood-stabilizing medications. Dr. Frank adds, "While patients need to lead more regular lives, that doesn't mean that they need to lead boring lives."

Michael Smolensky, Ph.D., of the University of Texas School of Public Health, is also examining the chronobiological relation to mood illness, especially depression. Dr. Smolensky has noticed that depressed patients typically awaken too early and have low activity in the morning; their early-morning mood coincides with their nightly biorhythms. Because their mood doesn't take off and rise until late morning or early afternoon, they experience low activation all around. In other words, certain patients' tendency for depression is linked to the dislocation of their chronobiological rhythm. They try to interact with others when their body is shut down.

Daniel F. Kripke, M.D., Chronobiologist from the University of California at San Diego, warns that disorders of the biological clock in normal healthy subjects can ultimately lead to affective disorders such as depression and mania. Why? For Dr. Kripke, the issue involves the circadian system's "phase advance" or "phase delay," both typically associated with mood disorders. Manics and elderly, depressed patients tend to be "phase advanced," that is, they wake up very early and go to bed very early. Young people in their teens and twenties, or patients with winter depression tend to be "phase delayed" — they have trouble falling asleep and trouble waking. Phase advance and delay, especially in today's competitive environment, can cause severe sleep disturbances that could surface as mood illness.

Solutions

If you're phase advanced, consider using evening bright light; if you're phase delayed, try using morning bright light. Maintain bedtimes and rising times that are set in stone. Not all mood illness is related to your circadian pacemaker. If you have a regular sleep/wake schedule and still suffer severe mood swings and have scored poorly on the test in Step 9, "Build Mental Capital," then you need to consult your physician to discuss diagnosis and possible treatment, including medication.

Problem #5: Depression

Some people believe that being sad most of the time is part of life. Nothing could be further from the truth. Too many people accept depression and a negative, tired, and unproductive mood when they don't have to.

Keep in mind, however, that just because you had a bad week does not mean you have depressive illness and need to take drugs. Scott Goldsmith, M.D., Clinical Assistant Professor of Psychiatry at the Weill Medical College of Cornell University, says, "A diagnosis of depression is more complicated than just feeling blue, although that certainly can be a part of it. It's more like wearing a pair of eyeglasses that makes everything seem less pleasurable and more hopeless, a feeling that can last weeks to years. What a trained clinician will look for is a variety of factors, including mood disturbances, self-esteem difficulties, sleep and/or weight changes, an inability to get pleasure from things, low energy, and changes in concentration. Before considering medications, it is important to consider any underlying medical conditions that could mimic depression. You also need to evaluate what's happening in the context of a person's life, as life stress can lead to symptoms similar to depression, or may even lead to a depressive episode. The good news is that newer forms of medications and therapies can be remarkably helpful."

Solutions

If you've been suffering from depression for much of your adult life, you should strongly consider year in, year out use of antidepressants. If you have been the victim of tragic events, you may want to consider antidepressants only long enough to get yourself back on your feet. In either case, have your family doctor consult with a psychopharmacologist before taking action.

More than 80 percent of those suffering from depressive illness can be treated successfully with modern medications, but those medications need to be individually tailored to your biology and brain wiring. Alexander Vuckovic, M.D., a psychiatrist at McLean Hospital in Belmont, Massachusetts, and an instructor in psychiatry at Harvard Medical School, compares some of the modern antidepressants: "You'll find, for example, that Prozac may have an energizing effect so that it is given to patients whose depression has slowed them down. Serzone, on the other hand, has more sedating properties for patients who suffer anxiety." Psychiatrists like my father have found that for moderate to severe depression the MAO (monoamine oxidase)-inhibitor class of drugs are the most power-ful and effective antidepressants. Whereas Paxil, for example, can take away the "edge" that may have been what made you successful, MAO inhibitors maintain the "edge" while giving your brain energy and powerful antidepressant action. Many doctors are fearful of the side effects when the antidepressants are taken with the wrong drugs, alcohol, or cheese (aged foods produce a substance called tyramine, which is normally broken down by MAO, so that when you inhibit MAO you can cause an elevation in blood pressure from too much tyramine). The biggest new trend in psychopharmacol-ogy is to take two drugs together, creating a synergistic effect. For instance, according to Dr. Vuckovic, Wellbutrin or Dexedrine may be given with SSRI (selective serotonin reuptake inhibitor) drugs such as Prozac or Paxil. Other doctors will add a small dose of thyroid hormone to an antidepressant for an energizing effect. Still others will combine two different categories of antidepressants, a tricyclic with a serotonin reuptake inhibitor. More and more researchers realize that we all have very different mood chemistries requiring strikingly different kinds of drugs. Certain drugs work very well within families. For example, if Paxil works for one mem-ber of the family, it's more likely to work for all members. These examples are not given as specific recommendations but to indicate the breadth of treatment choices available.

There are artificial cutoffs for frank depression at the low end and mania at the top end, but in between you are really free to choose where you would like to spend your life. I cannot believe the transformation in members of my own family and in patients whose mood reset to a higher level. Unfortunately, with the advent of managed care, fewer patients may have ready access to a psycho-pharmacologist. This leads to real mismatches between patient and drug. I have found that top psychopharmacologists are modern-day wizards who can concoct a mixture of different medications and hormones that perfectly suits your moods and personality.

The right drug can make or break your career. Manic-depressives have a long history of tremendous creativity. The long list of artists, musicians, and writers with manic-depression would almost make one believe the disease were a prerequisite for creative life. However, many manic-depressives will tell you that after being treated for both their mania and depression, they had the most productive years of their lives. That's why a highly accurate diagnosis and assessment by a top psychopharmacologist is key to deciding if you need medication and what kind you need. The pitfalls of not getting the right kind of help are legion.

Imagine a "personality pill" — in other words, harnessing the very most powerful drugs used in psychiatry, not to treat mental illness but to enhance performance. Can it work? A recent study showed that Paxil given to individuals with no psychiatric disease at all actually improved subtle aspects of their personality. At Allegheny General Hospital, a study is under way for what I call "terrible personality" syndrome. It is a study of those people with whom we work with who are irritable, short-tempered, unfriendly, and generally unpleasant to be around. The results show that with antidepressant treatment, the terrible personality goes away.

Quite frankly, however, if you don't have a real depressive illness, you'll find a drug's side effects may far outweigh its benefits. A normal-functioning person whose mood is low from inactivity, poor foods, and a lack of sleep will find the loss of libido and lethargy associated with antidepressants too much to tolerate. There's also debate as to whether certain medications destroy part of your ability to succeed. Here are several anecdotes. A top business magnate with attention deficit disorder (ADD) finds that the disorder actually allows him to shift quickly his attention and energy from one deal to the other. Without ADD, he might focus and succeed at a single business, but he wouldn't be able constantly to shift his attention and energy from one industry to another, the very shifts that had helped him to build a major conglomerate. Dr. Vuckovic cites another example of a highly functioning investment banker prescribed an SSRI antidepressant. Although the banker felt more relaxed than he could ever remember, he had also lost his drive to do business. Medication might cause fatigue and loss of energy, and that's why I'm such a strong believer in the measures for improving mental energy found in Part One of this book.

If you do not have a low mood, remember that life's events or even a change in season to cold raw winter days could lower it. I've noticed in my own life that in the winter months, if I allow my mood to fall, I don't shoot as high, fail to make the contacts I should, and even feel undeserving of talking to the person that I need to talk to. But when the positive mood comes back it is simply stunning — much better plans, loftier goals, and the ability to tackle them. In Part Two of this book you will read a great deal about creating positive thought. Positive thought can have on depression an effect as powerful as drugs.

Problem #6: Winter Blahs

Seasonal Affective Disorder (SAD) is a disease that affects people during the short dark days of winter, when the sun is hidden or appears only briefly for several months. SAD is the most extreme form of "winter blues." Sufferers exhibit the classical symptoms of depression: they have trouble getting out of bed in the morning, are quickly fatigued, have an increased appetite (particularly for sweets or other fattening foods), and often put on extra weight. Some sufferers sleep more and withdraw from social activities. Symptoms such as social withdrawal and unwanted weight can compound depression. Women often suffer more than usual from premenstrual syndrome. Because the indoor lighting provides only a small fraction of the light of the sun, people who work indoors throughout the day, or night workers who sleep through daylight hours, are especially vulnerable to SAD and indeed can experience SAD-like symptoms all year round.

Michael Terman, Ph.D., Professor of Clinical Psychology in Psychiatry at Columbia University, just concluded a six-year clinical trial, the longest and largest study ever conducted on light therapy. He compared four different treatment conditions:

- in the morning, upon awakening, exposure to a bright light of 10,000 lux for thirty minutes;

- in the evening, ninety minutes before sleeping, exposure to a bright light of 10,000 lux for thirty minutes;

- in the morning, upon awakening, exposure to high-density negative ions at the same time as bright light therapy;

- in the morning, upon awakening, exposure to a placebo control condition of low-density negative ions that are comparable to what one would get from a normal home air cleaner.

He discovered that both light treatments as well as high-density ion treatment were much more beneficial than the placebo treatment. Morning light was statistically the best; more people showed remission of depression under morning light than under any other condition. And when the light therapy was stopped, depression returned. But the big breakthrough for the rest of us is that extrinsic clinical observation and at least one formal research study have shown that intensive light therapy is effective for people with "winter doldrums," a milder version of SAD.*

Solutions

The kind and quality of light you have makes a big difference in how you feel. As mentioned earlier, buy a high-intensity light to ward off the winter blues. I use a high-intensity light attached to an artifical dawn simulator, so when it's a cold and dreary January in New York, I can wake up as if I were in Brazil.

If you suffer real symptoms of depression, you may want a light box in addition to your dawn simulator. Here's how the light therapy box works. Sit close to the light box containing a set of bright fluorescent bulbs hidden by a screen. Although researchers do not recommend looking at the light directly, you may interact freely with your surroundings during the light treatment. But use the light source to illuminate your activities. To get the maximum benefit of the light, it is very important that you sit with your head facing the light box, which is compatible with reading, and so on, but is not compatible with watching television. Even a small rotation of the

---

*Studies have shown that light therapy is effective not only for SAD but also for treating premenstrual disturbance and bulimia at any time of year. Administered in the second half of the month, light therapy can keep women free of PMS; and used regularly, light can markedly reduce the urge to binge eat.

head and eyes away from the frontal plane greatly reduces the amount of light that reaches the retina, and thus the treatment dose.

Sphere One (Web site: www.sphereone.com; phone: (212) 208-4438) provides the light boxes Dr. Terman used in his research. The Sphere One light therapy box delivers 10,000 lux illumination and is designed to remove ultraviolet light and to shine from above so that one doesn't look the light in the eye. If you have a retinal problem, you should not use bright light therapy without consulting an ophthalmologist and being monitored by a doctor.

Problem #7: Drugs That Keep You Awake

Certain drugs can delay the release of melatonin, the brain hormone that puts us to sleep. For example, patients often take arthritis drugs at bedtime in order to ease their next-day pain. These arthritis drugs, however, inhibit the release of melatonin, so by taking them at night you are disrupting your sleep cycle. In other words, from a chronobiological perspective, nighttime is actually the wrong time to take the arthritis drugs. A physician might prescribe you a sleep-enhancing drug, but before you take it, be careful to synchronize the medication with your biological needs. Using the right drug at the wrong time could aggravate the situation and cause you more sleepless nights.

Solutions

Review your medications with your doctor to determine which drugs may interfere with sleep. Remember, most illnesses keep their own biological clock and exhibit maximum symptoms at specific times of day, so plan carefully when to take your medications, and if possible, take sleep-killing drugs earlier in the day.

Problem #8: Fading Larks

"Morningness" and "eveningness" are terms used to describe a person's individual biological clock profile. We call "morning people" larks and "evening people" owls. Emmanuel Mignot, M.D., Ph.D., of the Stanford University Sleep Disorders Center in Palo Alto, California, suggests that these rhythms may be "hardwired." He reports that if you carry a distinct clock variant, called 3111C, you have "increased evening and decreased morning tendencies." He calculates that the average 3111C carrier has a "naturally programmed sleep time up to 44 minutes later than that of noncarriers." That means a person carrying the 3111C gene variant has the tendency to go to bed and wake up much later than someone without this variant.

Are you a lark or an owl? To find out, turn to the workbook and take the test graciously provided by J. A. Horne and O. Oestberg.

Morningness refers to early risers who typically prefer to rise between 5:00 A.M. and 7:00 A.M. and retire between 9:00 P.M. and 11:00 P.M.. There's a good reason why we call them larks: They're so cheery in the morning. In comparison to owls, when larks awake, they are a greater number of hours past their melatonin peak. In other words, larks are further from the last big dose of the body's internal sleeping medication, so they are naturally less groggy.

Researchers at Leiden University recently reported a finding explaining another biological difference between larks and owls. The researchers followed the body's daily temperature curve and found a time difference in the daily temperature curves of morning and evening people — larks had a biological clock that ran two hours earlier than owls.

The problem with being a lark is that you can fade fast through the afternoon and evening, losing many productive hours of work.

Solutions

If you're a lark, be sure to use the morning for maximum productivity. Try to get more out of your afternoons by eating a high-protein lunch and using exercise in the mid- to late afternoon to get another round of energy.

Problem #9: Grumpy Owls

Evening people or owls tend to prefer both a later wake-up (9:00 A.M.–11:00 A.M.) and a later bedtime (11:00 P.M.–3:00 A.M.). What determines an owl? Owls tend to have biological clocks set to "longer" days, around 24.8-hour days. That means that each morning, owls have a built-in tendency to oversleep. Owls have to get up at an earlier point in their biological rhythm in order to reset their circadian system by the amount of time that is needed to keep in sync with the twenty-four-hour day. When awakened, owls show a lower mood because they are rising at a time when their biological clocks are telling them to still be asleep. They go to bed on Eastern Standard Time, but want to wake up on Central or Rocky Mountain time. Owls would sleep until, say, 9:00 A.M. because that is what their biological rhythms are telling them to do. Unfortunately, they have the 7:00 A.M. wake-up call like everyone else, and that makes most owls grouchy and pretty unproductive in the morning.

Solutions

Owls can have the best of both worlds if they can recover their mornings. The key problem with owls is that they have a drive to keep going late into the evening. They chronically push the envelope on trying to stay up reading, writing, on the phone, watching TV. Owls benefit most by great sleep preparations and then forcing themselves to get up at the same time each morning and expose themselves to morning light. For sound sleep that provides optimal recovery, follow the guidelines provided earlier in this chapter.

Problem #10: Travel Sickness

Top sleep experts consider the severe lack of sleep caused by frequent travel to different time zones for short periods of time as an illness. In the news business, you can be in New York one day and Mozambique, Bangladesh, the Congo, or Kosovo the next. Mental performance sags miserably, and you may even feel nauseated as well as weak. It's hard to exercise or even organize your thoughts. That's because your geographic location is set at one time zone while your biological clock is at another. At noon in Tokyo, your biological clock is set for midnight, melatonin is putting you to sleep, your blood pressure and pulse are falling. Then when you try to fall asleep at 10:00 P.M. Tokyo time, all body systems are at full go, with loads of the hormones that get you going in the morning. All you can do is stare at the ceiling.

Solutions

Experts believe that to adjust your circadian rhythm, you require a day per hour of change in time zones. Older people, especially when flying against the sun, might well need 2 days per hour shift or time zone crossed. The biggest trouble with time travel comes from your body's internal time clock causing natural peaks and valleys in blood levels of key hormone levels such as thyroid or cortisol. If you're trying to sleep while these levels are high, you'll find your sleep disturbed and the next day ruined. As I write this page, I'm on a flight from Jeddah, Saudi Arabia, to New York, about to enter a time change of seven hours. In the old days I'd really suffer for days, fighting to think and with little motivation to work out. Now that I avoid alcohol or too much food and understand the proper use of light and sleep medication, my life on the road has been transformed.

MEDICATIONS

MELATONIN Melatonin has a half-life of only about an hour and a half, so that after an hour and a half the level of melatonin in your bloodstream has been reduced by 50 percent. That means melatonin is a very short-acting drug, and those who take this drug at 10:00 P.M. will have no problem falling asleep but they might well have problems staying asleep! If your problem is going to sleep, take it at bedtime; if your problem is waking in the middle of the night — well, take it then! But be careful. Melatonin tends to be overprescribed. It is not advisable to take melatonin during the day. By introducing melatonin in the day when it is never naturally used, you upset normal sleep patterns. MIT's Dr. Richard Wurtman recommends only 0.3 mg. Unfortunately, only a fortunate minority find that melatonin works well for them on long-haul flights. The rest of us may need stronger stuff.

SLEEPING PILLS I had long stayed away from medication, believing that sleeping pills were addictive and just plain bad for you. I've changed my mind. Finding the right sleep medication transforms time travel. For eastbound travel, I'll take a sleeping pill on takeoff and sleep as much of the flight as possible. Staying up for dinner and champagne will come back to haunt you the following day. Which sleeping pill works best is a matter of individual biology. Halcion has developed a particularly nasty reputation, yet there's almost nothing more likely to knock you down for the count during a long transoceanic flight. A new favorite is Ambien, which many travelers find to have fewer side effects. As with most medications, however, about 10 percent of the population experience unpleasant side effects or reactions to sleeping pills — so be careful. Discuss the pros and cons of sleeping pills with your doctor.

LIGHT

Body and brain temperature as well as melatonin hormone levels are important markers of your biological clock. The body and brain are warmer during the day than during the night; and melatonin levels are very low during the day and high during the night. Dr. Derk-Jan Dijk, Assistant Professor of Medicine at Harvard Medical School, says that these variations correlate with performance. We perform better during the day than during the night. The timing of these rhythms in temperature, hormones, and performance can be reset by scheduled exposure to light. When you're traveling, make sure you go to bed and wake up at the local time. And once awake in the morning, go out into the sunlight — this allows the sun to reset your biological time clock. If it's winter and dark outside, turn on all the indoor lights to help you reset your clock.

CHOOSING FLIGHTS

WEST TO EAST Going from the United States to Europe, try for a daylight flight if it is offered. Keep the window shade up and try to stay awake for the entire flight. If you have to take a night flight, take a flight early enough in the evening to get a great night's sleep and wake up with the dawn. For overnight flights, try to stay in the dark as long as possible by selecting flights that leave early in the evening, say 6:00 instead of 11:00. Rather than connecting flights, try to get a direct flight long enough to get a full night's rest. For instance, instead of flying Boston-London-Cairo, you're better off flying first to New York then getting a nonstop to Cairo. You'll get eight hours of uninterrupted sleep, instead of five to England, then have to wake up, walk to the next plane, and try to sleep fitfully on the way to Cairo.

If you're only staying for a few days in a new time zone, keep your watch set on your home time zone and try if at all possible not to stray too far from your home time zone. If you've left New York and are in Europe for two days, go to bed at, say, 2:00 A.M. and get up at 9:00 A.M. or 10:00 A.M., so you're close to Eastern Standard Time. If your flight arrives at 7 A.M., wear very dark glasses until 10.00 A.M., so you don't reset your clock. When you are sleeping in the next morning, be sure to keep your room dark so that you don't reset your clock.

EAST TO WEST Always fly with the sun — that is, while the sun is up rather than at night. Since your body's time clock resets faster flying west, use the sun to your advantage. Try to keep your aircraft window shade open. When you arrive, stay up until the sun goes down.

Whenever you encounter a problem with your biological clock, return to this chapter. Remember, "normal" for different people relates in part to our social and cultural experience of mornings and evenings. One hundred fifty years ago, for instance, when almost everyone had a cow that needed to be milked, it was common to rise at 4:00 A.M.! Today it's not. Today, a regular sleep schedule might mean going to sleep at 10:00 P.M. and waking up at 6:00 A.M. If you can't get to bed until 2:00 in the morning and can't rise before 10:00, you could lose your job.

Many of us underestimate what a tremendous power our pacemakers have for alertness and mental energy. That's because many of us haven't dusted off our pacemakers in years. With your ECP brightened and mental energy at a new high level, you'll be ready for Part Two, "Create Positive Thought."

PART TWO

——— |||||| ———

Create Positive Thought

Introduction

In Part One, we learned how to create massive amounts of mental energy. But in and of itself, mental energy does not equal success. A lab rat could have great mental energy. What the lab rat doesn't have and a human being does is a large cerebral cortex, the thinking part of the brain that makes genius possible. In theory, you could make a complete idiot quite energetic and happy, as evidenced by classic comics from the Three Stooges to Laurel and Hardy. Mental energy is only a platform, a launching pad for positive thought. It is in the cerebral hemispheres where positive thinking and creative thought occur that life's grand successes are born. Part Two, "Create Positive Thought," will help you gear your mental drive to its highest limits.

CONVENTIONAL WISDOM: Don't worry, be happy.

THE BIOLOGY OF SUCCESS: Light up the sky.

The Biology of Positive Thought

A whole new school of psychiatry has grown up around the development of positive thinking. The key is intercepting negative thoughts. Surprisingly, no matter how positive we think we are, many of us have internal, mostly negative chatter that ties up the cerebral circuits all day long. Much of this chatter is actually pretty idiotic if you stop and listen to it. Most of the time we're simply ripping ourselves apart. The more negative our mood, the more we're apt to nag ourselves. The science of positive thought can be learned through certain therapies, of which cognitive therapy is one example.

Cognitive therapy teaches you to catch the negative thoughts in this gnawing pitter-patter and substitute much more reasonable, reassuring, and, most important, more accurate thoughts. During cognitive therapy, the therapist uses various techniques of talk therapy and behavioral prescriptions to help the patient alleviate and change his or her negative thought patterns and beliefs. For example, a salesman fails to get through to an account on a sales call and actually encounters a very rude rebuff from the secretary. His inner voice might say, "See, you're no damned good, never were." He'd do better to catch that negative thought, judge it, and turn it into a more accurate reply such as: "Gee it was early and the secretary must have had a bad night. Her boss probably had a bad night too and she was taking it out on me. I'm actually a pretty good salesperson; I'll just try again at a better time of day." This is cognitive therapy at work.

Part Two of this book contains six powerful steps for developing positive thinking, but before we turn to them, let's take a closer look at cognitive therapy as proof of the concept that positive thought does truly change the brain.

Cognitive Therapy

Cognitive therapy is based on the theory that people's emotions are controlled by their views and opinions of the world. Depression results when patients constantly berate themselves, expect to fail, make inaccurate assessments of what others think of them, feel hopeless, and have a negative attitude toward the world and the future.

You may think that "talk" therapy is all vaporware, but consider this. Using the gold standard PET scan, researchers noticed that patients who engaged in cognitive therapy had changes just as marked on the PET scan as patients taking Prozac. This shows that positive thinking on its own can change the way your brain functions, a true revolution in modern psychiatry. This "talk therapy" can be at least as good as drugs. Why? First, after repeated talk therapy, new and important connections are created between one set of neurons and another. That means that your brain is fundamentally, even if ever so slightly, changing. Second, even without drugs, cognitive therapy increases levels of neurotransmitters that battle depression and anxiety.

Cognitive therapy *can* change the brain circuitry, concludes Richard Davidson, Ph.D., after reviewing hard data. For example, it's been shown that in obsessive-compulsive behavior, cognitive therapy can produce changes in circuitry — actual biological changes in the brain.

Susan C. Vaughan, M.D., convinced of the effectiveness of talk therapy, has written a book named after Freud's phrase, *The Talking Cure*. "Talking changes the structure of the brain itself; the nerve cells end up with different connections so they grow differently and the new connections form new structures. It is through the change in connections that you learn and that's how you store information; that's how you make links between cells that weren't connected before and there's knowledge in that link," Dr. Vaughan says. So talking makes new connections between brain cells; experience changes the shape of and connections between brain cells. The cerebral cortex and the association cortex (in the parietal lobes) are mainly implicated in "talk therapy"; those are the highest level of cortex — they put together the most information from that part of the brain. After several years of psychotherapy, the brain may look different; but because changes are occurring between neurons, at a very small cell-to-cell level, they're hard to see. Still, these cerebral cortex changes are longer lasting than medications because you're changing the structure of your brain, whereas medication is only changing brain chemistry. In treatment of depression, the best results are achieved with a combination of drugs and psychotherapy, because the two are synergistic.

The Argument for Complex Thought

A new publishing industry has grown up around the concept of dumbing down complex ideas. One sees that in many aspects of life in America, where nearly everything has to be nugget-sized and simple, from our basic foods to our music. The dumbing-down effect would have us watching *Seinfeld* reruns instead of plowing through important new technological information, philosophical argument, or historical texts that could improve our minds and further our career. Our approaches to diet and exercise are so timid that it's a wonder we're not all hopelessly overweight and out of shape. This great timidity in America is transforming us into a nation of lemmings. There is a much broader world out there — not one that is more intimidating, just more rewarding, a world that challenges us to master greater complexity.

Simply put, the greatest joy in life can be undertaking and mastering complex activities such as learning a new language or listening to and understanding a symphony or studying the classics or mastering an unfamiliar historical period. In Part One of the book, we looked at all the comparatively simple ways of improving mood and brain energy. No one, however, wants to be the happy fool. In fact many believe that happiness is a nonattainable condition . . . that we can never be free of yearnings and anxieties. But we can achieve great satisfaction by developing the positive thought that encourages us to tackle complex tasks and succeed. That hard work pays off quickly.

As we master complex thoughts and develop greater successes, work actually becomes far easier. Fran Shea says: "At the beginning of my career I spent a huge number of hours at work. I could spend up to fifteen hours a day working. But I was absolutely in love with my job. There was nothing about my job I didn't like. I had way more ideas than I could fulfill. I was lucky. I was in a business that was booming. I was there at the right time." Now she is president of E! Entertainment Networks and one of the top women in broadcasting. Dr. Richard J. Haier, of the Department of Pediatrics at the University of California at Irvine, has used brain imaging to measure brain activity and metabolism. The student subjects in his laboratory were tested at the video game Tetris. These students were scanned during the first day of practice, when they showed great metabolic activity. They were scanned again after two months of practice. Although the subjects had increased their abilities sevenfold, the scans showed their metabolic activity to have lessened dramatically. So the study showed that the more gifted we become at something, the fewer circuits in the brain we use. In other words, we're able to do the same activity with less effort. While Tetris is not a sophisticated or complex mental activity, the experiment does show that success in conquering mental complexities is a case of the brain working smarter, not harder.

In the following chapters, we'll look at specific steps to build a strong pattern of positive thought. Here's a brief road map.

Step 1: Be an Optimist

Learn the heart of a positive mental attitude by transforming yourself into a tough-minded optimist. This is rigorous science, not pop psychology.

Step 2: Seize the Moment

Shed your anxieties and the distractions that pull you from success by learning the skills of accomplished actors and committing fully to the moment at hand.

Step 3: Play to Your Strengths

Take a unique test to determine the way your personality is wired. Then learn to use that knowledge to relate better to others. Learn how to chase success based on how your brain is wired.

Step 4: Learn Emotional Broadcasting

By learning emotional broadcasting, learn to convert those around you to allies who will give you the emotional support and team strength you need to succeed. "Emotional Broadcasting" is the "networking" of the twenty-first century, literally changing the emotions of those around you.

Step 5: Look to the Hereafter

Learn prayer to gain an even greater sense of optimism and positive thought. As with optimism, the new interest in spirituality is based on firm scientific studies.

Step 6: Create a Blueprint for Success

This final step will help you channel and focus all your mental energy and positive thought into creating and embodying your life's story.

Step 1:
Be an Optimist

||||||

OK, so maybe you hate optimists. You have this picture in your mind of someone mindlessly watching *Pollyanna* on the late show until three o'clock in the morning, then rising at 5:00 A.M. and singing "Zip-a-Dee-Doo-Dah" in the shower until the entire household is awake, causing a bad start to an otherwise perfectly OK day. A far more discerning look at optimists shows that they are life's big winners. They are richer, more successful, healthier, do better in school, and have both better relationships and marriages. Linda S. Wilson, President Emerita of Radcliffe, says: "I'm an optimist. Optimism is the expectation that we can make things better. For example, in the face of pending illness, assume that it has the probability of coming out OK. It's important not to have a defeatist attitude." What's different about optimists is that they are tough-minded and creative when faced with adversity. Optimism is high mental energy. Fran Shea, President of E! Entertainment, says: "I think optimism is something you have to put effort into. I'm optimistic by nature, but society is so sped up, and that contributes to the overwhelm mode. Not having time to prioritize works against optimism."

> **CONVENTIONAL WISDOM:** Optimists can't handle reality.

> **THE BIOLOGY OF SUCCESS:** Optimists are the most skillful manipulators of reality.

The Biology of Optimism

Individuals who are more optimistic report themselves to be more alert, more proud, more enthusiastic, active, and engaged. These individuals are less likely to get depressed. Dr. Richard J. Davidson, Professor of Psychology and Psychiatry at the University of Wisconsin–Madison, has studied the biology of optimism and found optimists have higher levels of natural killer-cell activity with a smaller decline under stress, so they are more capable of fighting disease. Optimists also have lower levels of the stress hormone cortisol. All these observations add up to solid biological advantages that may help explain why optimists are generally so much more successful than pessimists.

Creating the Biology of Optimism

Much of what follows in this section is born of conversations with Professor Martin Seligman, Ph.D., author of the acclaimed bestseller *Learned Optimism* and the world's leading authority on optimism, helplessness, and explanatory styles.

Overcoming helplessness

The number one stumbling block to reaching success for most people is that they do not genuinely believe that they can succeed. They have learned, over time, how to become helpless. This condition, which Dr. Seligman calls "learned helplessness," is at the very heart of pessimism. We invent a million different excuses as to why we can't do something — and you know what . . . as a result we can't. The sad truth is that we are creating our own flawed destiny through pessimism. Dr. Seligman says pessimism is a self-fulfilling prophecy: "Twenty-five years of study have convinced me that if we habitually believe that misfortune is our fault, is enduring, and will undermine everything we do, more of it will befall us than if we believe otherwise. . . . If we are in the grip of this view, we will get depressed easily, we will accomplish less than our potential, and we will even get physically sick more often. Pessimistic prophecies are self-fulfilling." Pessimists are more passive and less likely to take steps to avoid bad events and less likely to do anything to stop them once they start.

Who are you? Are you an optimist or a pessimist? Which category do you fall into? The typical pessimist believes that when something bad happens, it will last a long time, that the event has undermined everything he's ever done, that it's entirely his fault. The pessimist imagines the worst, is prone to depression, and generally feels helpless. The optimist believes that a bad event is temporary and surmountable, that it's a cause of bad luck or other people. The optimist is unfazed by defeat and feels the bad event is a challenge to overcome. He or she easily regains energy and above all feels in control. How you explain life's events to yourself determines if you are an optimist or pessimist. For pessimists, those events are explained by Professor Seligman's three "p's" of pessimism.

PERMANENCE

Pessimists give up easily because they believe the situation is permanent. The bad events will continue and always be a part of their lives. An optimist believes the causes of bad events are temporary. Here's an example you may find in your own relationships:

> PESSIMIST: "You never talk to me."
> OPTIMIST: "You haven't talked to me lately."

When things go wrong, everyone experiences a momentary sense of failure. How quickly you bounce back is reflective of this dimension of permanence.

PERVASIVENESS

Some people let failure pervade every aspect of their lives. If you lose your job, your role as a wife or a daughter or a volunteer has not diminished one bit. Dr. Seligman says it comes down to this: universal versus specific explanations. "People who make universal explanations for their failures give up on everything when a failure strikes in one area. People who make specific explanations may become helpless in that one part of their lives yet march stalwartly on in the others."

PERSONALIZATION

Whom do you blame when something goes wrong? Those who internalize blame tend to have low self-esteem, feeling unloved or unworthy, while the opposite is true for those who place the blame outside themselves.

Becoming an optimist

This section will take you, step by step, toward being an optimist. The more optimistic you become, the more your mood will lift.

Becoming an optimist means learning a set of skills that help you to talk to yourself when you confront failure, a setback, or a tragedy. You'll do that by changing the way you explain events to yourself. Technically, Dr. Seligman calls it the ABCDE (Adversity, Belief, Consequence, Disputation, Energization) method. Here's an example of how to fight pessimistic thoughts by changing the way you explain bad events.

ADVERSITY

You've gotten up at the crack of dawn, made the beds, called two new clients, and are about to leave for work when your four-year-old flips his breakfast onto the floor. You totally lose it and scream at the little tyke, who gives you a look of bewilderment.

BELIEF

"I'm a lousy mother. I just can't do it all. I'm providing a miserable example of how to behave and can't even be nice to my own children. My children will grow up to be hostile people who deal with the world through the prism of anger and frustration. They'll never amount to much of anything."

CONSEQUENCE

"I'm depressed."

DISPUTATION

A good way to dispute any charge is to imagine that your worst enemy said that to you. You wouldn't believe that you were a lousy mother and would argue the point SO, ARGUE! Like a lawyer launching an attack on a hostile witness, prepare the following arguments to counter your pessimistic thought.

- Make your belief factually incorrect with evidence. Look at all the evidence showing you that in fact you're not a lousy mother — you take good care of your children, get them to school on time, read to them . . . you just had a bad moment.

- Decatastrophize the implications of the situation. OK, you yelled. Just how bad is that? Does that mean your child won't graduate from Harvard or will become an ax murderer? Yelling once is just not a catastrophe.

- Search for alternative explanations for your behavior. Focus on the causes that are changeable, specific, and nonpersonal. For instance, you were up all night with a new baby and just felt a little cranky. That's a long way from being a bad mother.

- Look at the usefulness of your belief. How useful or productive is it for you to think you're a lousy mother? Does that really help you be a better mother? Often, it's simply better to get on with what you have to do, to distract yourself, than to dwell on destructive beliefs.

ENERGIZATION

Now pick yourself up, dust yourself off, and start to feel good about yourself. Take a lesson from Step 4, "Practice Emotional Broadcasting," and have a chat with the poor little guy. Help him dispute feeling badly about himself. Tell him accidents do happen and that he's a great little guy. Provide a real emotional bond. Try the same thing when you get into an altercation with adults. Let the anger cool, then try to change the emotional atmosphere so that you are energized by the situation and walk away feeling better for having undergone it.

Once you change your explanatory style from pessimistic to optimistic, research suggests that the change is permanent. You will have set skills for talking to yourself when you fail. You can use these skills to stop depression from taking hold when failure strikes. On a philosophical level, changing explanatory styles works because, as Dr. Seligman says, "it takes advantage of newly legitimized powers of the self." For more help, you'll want to read Professor Seligman's excellent book, *Learned Optimism*. The ADAPTIV company now makes his methods more widely available to businesses. For further help, you may also seek out psychiatrists or psychologists who practice cognitive therapy.

Immunizing against Pessimism

The late Jonas Salk, M.D., the polio vaccine pioneer, told me, "If I were a young scientist today, I would still do immunization. But instead of immunizing kids physically, I would do it psychologically. I'd see if these psychologically immunized kids could then fight off mental and physical illness better."

Seligman proved this psychological immunization could work through an elegant animal experiment. You may recall the classic Pavlovian experiment in which rats learned to avoid electric shocks by discovering what actions caused the shock. What Professor Seligman did was to take rats that had thoroughly mastered the art of avoiding electric shocks, and then put these animals in a situation in which they could not avoid the shock. Because they had been "immunized" against helplessness, the rats continued to avail themselves of every imaginable effort to avoid the new series of shocks. They had learned how to help themselves and weren't about to give up. They were optimistic rats. However, rats who could not escape the series of electric shocks in their early training learned how to become helpless or pessimistic. They simply wouldn't move no matter how painful or often the shocks.

Does the immunization of optimism work against real human illness? Consider these two studies.

A classic study at Harvard Medical School followed Harvard graduates for fifty years after they graduated, permitting a rare opportunity to follow the effect of positive thinking over an entire lifetime. Those who handled life with humor, altruism, and positive thinking went on to much more successful and healthy lives. By sixty, very few of them were chronically ill. Fully one-third of those who were pessimistic in their thinking showed poor health by age sixty.

In a groundbreaking study, David Spiegel, M.D., Director of the Psychosocial Treatment Laboratory at Stanford University School of Medicine, showed that women suffering from breast cancer lived eighteen months longer than their counterparts if they participated in weekly groups that involved strong social support and encouraged expression of all emotion — positive and negative. Dr. Spiegel says, "These groups developed realistic optimism — members learned to hope for the best but prepare for the worst. We found that when these women with advanced breast cancer shared their grief, sadness, and fear together, they also shared great joy. They learned to trivialize the trivial in their lives and value their contact with one another, their families, and friends." With a better social support system, the patients fared better; they learned that expressing honest emotion is a source of closeness with others, and that, in turn, made them feel better. The good news is that in this study, it wasn't innate optimism that was associated with living longer, it was developing a positive attitude and participating in a group that made them feel that they — and all of their emotions about the illness — belonged. Even in the face of insurmountable obstacles, such as death itself, optimists triumph. Says Dr. Spiegel, "The lesson is to focus on facing the illness directly, understanding that you can live richly even if you are dying of breast cancer."

Tommy Lasorda, the famous baseball coach, once told me that if you've got a great attitude, you've got a chance — with a bad attitude, you've got nothing. I'm amazed that more and more people today have a major attitude problem. Those who stand out as successes in their profession usually have a great attitude. In fact, a great attitude is probably the most important part of making your own good luck. That great attitude is what gets you noticed by people who *want* to hire you and work with you. Too many people with a bad attitude are tinged by just enough pessimism that many of the rest of us want to keep them at arm's length in order not to be infected by their negativity.

A bad attitude becomes a self-fulfilling prophecy. The individual with a bad attitude believes the events that have soured his attitude are out of his control, and that as a result he is damaged goods. When optimistic, you fundamentally believe something is possible. Optimists may get knocked around a lot, their ideas may get trashed, their careers thwarted, but by getting up instead of knocking their heads against the wall, they win again and again. Dr. Michael DeBakey, the famed heart surgeon, did bypass surgeries five years before they were proven effective, established the link between smoking and lung cancer in 1937, and was the first doctor to back Medicare. In each case he found himself awash in criticism. How did he pull through? "I think *optimism* is the basic attitude." Optimism, a basic belief in himself, and self-discipline. Dr. DeBakey adds self-discipline because it is the belief in self tied together with self-discipline that allows one to be optimistic in the face of adversity.

Many of us do have doubts about ourselves, about our abilities, or even about the feasibility of our life's work. If you're pessimistic, you'll never believe you can do anything, and that will leave you without a chance. Remember, even the wildest optimists sometimes fail in the scope of their vision. But look back through the long lens of history. Man almost always *under*estimated what could be done. Alexander Graham Bell most likely never foresaw cell phones or low earth-orbiting satellites for worldwide sat phone operations. Rather than envisioning something too grand, we imagine too little.

The bottom line is that optimism is the foundation of positive thoughts. By becoming optimistic, you remove the energy-draining funnel of pessimism. Consider the author Frederick Langbridge's epigram titled "Pessimist and Optimist":

> Two men look out through the same bars:
> One sees the mud, and one the stars.

Look out and see the stars! The more optimistic you are the greater your chances of remaining vibrantly healthy, beating disease, living longer, being more successful at work, having a better marriage, and becoming far more financially secure.

Step 2: Seize the Moment

———— |||||||| ————

Happiness, motivation, peak performance, and energy come when we're living in the moment. Jon Niednagel, Director of the Brain Type Institute in California and an expert in how the brain works to regulate mental and physical performance, says, "Happiness will come when we're more or less just perceiving life, enjoying it, and relaxing." How can you do this? "Stop analyzing everything. People need to loosen up and be involved not so much in the results, but the process." We all perform our best when we get involved in the process and enjoy the process. Take as an example a conversation you are having with a friend or colleague. How annoying it is when you don't get her full undivided attention. Her eyes look in a different direction, she fidgets, checks somebody else out. She really isn't listening to what you're saying but is preparing to launch into her own monologue, almost unaware of your thoughts or feelings. That friend or colleague should be concentrating on exactly what is happening in that moment. She should be caught up in perceiving that moment in time, focusing on what you are saying, how you are saying it, the emotion of the moment. The mistake many of us make is in ignoring the moment. By doing so we really hold the present off at arm's length. We stand back from it and ponder it rather than participating in it. Nowhere is that more exasperating or evident than in a conversation. A great conversationalist is totally caught up in what you are saying, understands what it is you are communicating, feels your emotion, and then reacts in a natural and empathetic way. When someone is preparing his own rebuttal during the time you are talking, he escapes the moment and misses whatever you may be communicating. I notice this is especially true in television journalism. You will see an interviewer fidgeting with cards, listening on an earpiece to a producer, preparing the next question . . . anything but listening to the interviewee's answer. The very best interviewers are totally caught up in what their subject is saying. That's what's so innocent and charming about Katie Couric's style of television. She doesn't pretend to be interested, she is. She senses how you feel. Oprah Winfrey completely blocks out the technical aspects of television in order to enter completely into the moment. During a recent show I explained to her how white flour, white potatoes, white rice, and white bread increase blood sugar levels whereas brown rice and black beans maintain a healthfully lower blood sugar. Now most TV personalities would be quickly moving onto the next point, reading a cue card, looking at the monitor, checking time cues. Oprah, totally in the moment, turned to me and said, "So what you're saying, Doctor Bob, is that white is bad, white is bad and brown and black are good," to the delight of her audience.

> **CONVENTIONAL WISDOM:** Worry.
> **THE BIOLOGY OF SUCCESS:** Life is a command performance. Live in the moment.

The Biology of Being in the Moment

When you relax in the moment, you are priming the most creative part of your brain, the visualization center in the posterior part of the brain. You supercharge your creative thinking by turning on these visualization centers. It's not clear why that is, but the observation is right there in living Technicolor. When you relax in the moment, the PET scan lights these centers of visual thought. What scientists believe happens is that when we live entirely in the moment, we free up the brain to think visually by turning off parts of the brain that drain energy away into neurotic and anxious thinking. When you see a great movie, opera, ballet, or sports event, you become totally absorbed in the moment, with your visual centers glowing brightly as the anxious concerns of the day take a rest. It is one of life's great ironies: We believe we accomplish so much by constantly worrying, when in reality we are preventing ourselves from opening the most magnificent part of the brain, the center of visual thought. Thomas G. West, who has written an excellent book on visual thinking, *In the Mind's Eye,* says that many of the great thinkers in history thought visually — physicists Albert Einstein, Michael Faraday, and James Clerk Maxwell are but a few. Many experts believe that visual thinking is the highest form of intelligence. Great athletes also think visually. They live exclusively in the moment and it pays off in Olympic Gold.

For the rest of us who are not Olympians, it is just as critical to strip away energies that are going in any direction but in the moment so that we can light up this most creative part of our brain. Many of us are so preoccupied with what we're going to do next or what terrible misfortune may befall us or what has already befallen us that we simply fail to operate fully and at our best in the moment. Many people fail to live in the moment because they believe that if you live FOR the moment you will lose your grasp on reality. That's not what being IN the moment means. If you truly want to grasp the opportunity that is laid in front of you at any given moment, you should be consumed by the moment.

How to Enter the Moment

Become an actor or actress

The very best actors in the world succeed by becoming bold and brave enough to exist only in the moment. You can acquire these same skills. You may think that's completely wrong because actors and actresses are "faking" it. However, the very best never fake anything. They are absolutely true to every word that comes out of their mouth. Why? Because they are living totally in the moment, living the lines they are speaking as they speak them. Here's how you can practice.

READ ALOUD

The best and most practical way of practicing how to be in the moment is to read aloud. Try reading aloud on a daily basis. The key is to truly own the material. Glance at it, lift it off the page, and just say it. Don't dramatize the line. Think of lines as thoughts or images and let the line do the talking. Say it as if it were a real conversation and you're the one speaking. Reading aloud will immediately get you to think, act, and be in the moment. If you have children or a spouse, read to them. Or volunteer your time to read to the sick in the hospital — a great way to escape your own troubles and dive into the moment.

Harold Guskin is the most famous acting coach in New York, teaching stars such as Kevin Kline, Glenn Close, and Bridget Fonda. First and foremost, he will teach you not to "do" anything with the words that you read. By just saying the words as they hit you, you'll find that your mind colors the words in a wonderful way. Take Robert De Niro as an example. He often speaks in the most understated manner possible. His voice, however, is still exploding with color and meaning. Being in the moment is what matters. Harold says: "It is an exploration of the moment without concern for where the moment is going. One's concentration should not be on how to do something or how to say it but rather on what it is and what it means. For an actor, if you think about how you're going to do something or how you're going to say it, you will manipulate the way you say it and it will sound contrived. You want it to sound like a human being so the audience can forget that you're an actor on stage. Even if what you're saying is effectively contrived, you will still seem false or 'actorish' — or like an 'old-fashioned actor.' The key is to say what you mean without trying to fix it up. What you say must be more important than *how* you say it."

You may say, "My life isn't a goddamn Bruce Willis movie! It's real life. How can this advice help me?" Well, Harold's advice has to do with courage, trust, and fear, traits most of us, including actors, have trouble with. Once you have mastered reading aloud in the moment, carry these techniques into conversations with friends and relatives, then colleagues at work. You'll be amazed how useful this skill will be in meetings with your boss or coworkers, dinner dates, or gatherings with your family. Rather than rambling, you'll be talking and listening to others as if there were nothing else going on in the universe, and as a result, all of your interactions will become more fresh and alive and you'll suddenly find yourself much more attractive to others.

Here's how you can incorporate Harold's advice into your everyday life: Concentrate on each word you say as you say it. Block out all other thoughts. Don't try to monitor yourself or think ahead. Most of us try to prepare the next couple of sentences, but that makes us extremely dull and predictable. When you look at a really great talent, say David Letterman, he literally doesn't know where he's going next because he's exploring the moment. That's what makes him so unexpectedly funny. You will be amazed how creative you really are when you just allow the next thought to come. Be assured that it really will come and will be far more interesting than whatever rote statements, stories, or jokes you might have prepared. The breakthrough in my own career on live television and public speaking was having the courage to just let the next thought come rather than preparing rote answers. This allowed for the unexpected and made me much fresher and more interesting than if I simply rattled off a bunch of facts. You'll be amazed at how much more positive and natural an impression you'll make. When you do thinking work, such as writing a proposal or reading a document, try to be totally in the moment so that you are consumed by what you're writing or reading. Read it aloud. Allow yourself to read and reread it aloud to find innovative solutions to problems you thought were insoluble.

Learn selflessness

Become totally absorbed in the moment by performing acts of such utter selflessness that you forget yourself. Consider this scene at the hospital in Baidoa, Somalia, in 1992: Our CBS News crew could hear the rat-a-tat-tat of automatic weapons fire in the marketplace, only a hundred yards away. Within minutes, bodies were thrown onto the floor of the makeshift emergency room run by an American group, the International Medical Corps. Twenty died before anything could be done. Among the forty remaining, there was a small four-year-old girl. She was clearly "bleeding out." There was no blood bank, no blood substitute. One doctor, a pediatrician named Mickey Richer, from Denver, Colorado, calmly took a intravenous needle, asked a technician to insert it into her vein, and then drew a pint of her own blood. She transfused her universal donor "O" positive blood into the small girl and saved her life.

Heroism is an act of utter selflessness, and it is only through heroic acts that I believe we become truly great. While you may never have the opportunity of jumping into a swift river to pull out a small child or running into a blazing building to drag out a trapped family, you do on a daily basis have the opportunity of practicing the same form of selflessness as front-page heroes. Those small acts of kindness go a very long way.

Many of us believe that Karma is some kind of good or bad will that indiscriminately afflicts us. In Buddhism, however, good Karma is built task by task. In a lecture I attended, Geshe Michael Roach of the Asian Classics Institute in New York emphasized that we are not made or broken by life's big events, but by how well we perform the mundane small tasks. How you say hello, your politeness in traffic, your helpfulness at work — each task is building either good or bad Karma. Perform tasks with a high mood, good spirits — in other words, with positive affect — and you will create your own good luck. Undertake them with resentment, anger, or negative affect, and you'll slowly sow the seeds of your own destruction. One of my father's patients, who had built a large fortune from nothing, explained his success by saying: "Don't spoil your success. The surest way to spoil your success is by littering your day with small acts of meanness."

Create a vision and then enter into it

Entering the moment unlocks your visual imaging capabilities in the posterior part of your brain. And remember, the strongest, most creative thought processes in the human brain are called visual spatial, basically thinking in three-dimensional pictures instead of words. According to Thomas West, when Einstein developed the theory of relativity, he did so by imagining it. Great poets such as William Butler Yeats imagined what they would write about, creating a picture, then putting it into words. Churchill was a visual thinker, as are many leaders of the new digital age. The reason that visual thinking is so important to positive thinking is that it allows you to run movies in your head. The more you run these movies, the less you'll focus on petty concerns that drag you out of the moment. I tell my son to enter the moment in a conversation by forming a mental image and then describing it, as a sports announcer describes a play. You'll find that you become much more alive in conversation than if you just grope for words. Describing a picture in your head concentrates your brain in the moment. Practice creating those visions during your afternoon nap or as you fall asleep at night. It's a great way to enter the present, forget the anxieties of the day, and put yourself to sleep.

Fight to stay in the present!

There are many forces dragging us out of the present. By monitoring exactly where you are, fight getting pulled into the past or the future. Below are two mottos to live by:

Don't let the future ruin the present. The greatest setback to living in the moment is having permanent anxiety about the future. For many of us, a hypothetical future ruins the present. I see this in the playground in New York. Amazing little children running, skipping, jumping, and playing in the playground while their fathers are standing by, cell phone in hand, oblivious to the great joy they could share with their children. Deeply anxious about the future, the fathers are busy making Saturday-morning phone calls to the office; rather than living in the moment and recovering from a long week of hard work, they're tense.

Don't get dragged into the past. Don't let the past ruin the present, either. Every small hurt and slight during a day, or a bigger one in the recent past, can find us replaying the event over and over. The setback could be missing a flight, getting a larger-than-expected credit card bill, denting a fender, spilling a drink, or losing a cell phone. If you've suffered an insult or setback, you want to get over it and quickly get back into the present. Try quickly to focus on what went wrong, why it went wrong, what you can do to prevent it in the future, and then instantly recover your good mood.

So seize each important moment of every day and live it to the fullest.

Step 3: Play to Your Strengths

———— |||||| ————

What if you want to think more positively but don't feel like becoming a big yahoo who screams through the halls beating his chest? A lot of thinking positively depends on knowing *how* to. If you're a true extrovert, you may really act out when you feel great. But if you're an introvert, you may want to keep it inside and push that quiet energy in a different direction. Einstein didn't look like a party animal, but you could see the power of positive thinking break through in his quiet smile, bright countenance, and sparkling eyes. You may feel like a wallflower when put up against a savvy, superpositive, high-charged salesman. You may also wonder how you could ever be like that person — smooth, polished, dazzling, and LOUD! Fundamental to understanding how to become successful is understanding how your brain is wired. If you are an introvert, that does not mean you can't have a positive thinking style and become extremely successful; it simply means that you will express it differently from an extrovert. Introversion and extroversion are the most commonly known of many key personality traits in the rapidly expanding field called psychological typology, which analyzes personality types. Understanding all of the traits will give you a dramatically improved ability to chase success. Until recently we didn't know how much of your particular type was determined by luck, personal development, environment, or actual brain wiring. Now researchers are beginning to link personality traits to brain scans and even specific genes. Neuroscience shows us that our brains are all wired differently. That means there can be no one stock path to success nor any overarching goals that will define success for everyone. The kind of success you will want to explore is based on how your brain is wired. Radcliffe President Emerita Linda S. Wilson says: "There are many different routes for success. I have respect for diversity in cognitive styles. I believe that we have failed to tap human potential because we have tried to find single blueprints instead of multiple blueprints." In this chapter, you'll find how to harness the strength of your brain type for your particular climb toward success.

> **CONVENTIONAL WISDOM:** Pour enough energy at somebody and you'll win them over.
> **THE BIOLOGY OF SUCCESS:** "To thine own self be true." Target your success based on brain type.

Many of us bang our heads against the walls trying to be something or someone we can't and might never really want to be. How many of us want to assume the personality of the highly successful Donald Trump or Leona Helmsley? Maybe we want their bank accounts and fame, but what about their personalities? Here's a brief look at testing personality traits and a surprisingly simple do-it-yourself test. Understanding your personality type and that of others is the key to the next Step, "Practice Emotional Broadcasting."

The MBTI Test

The Myers-Briggs Type Indicator (MBTI®) was developed by an American mother-and-daughter team, Katharine Briggs and Isabel Myers, and is based on the work of Carl Jung, the Swiss psychiatrist who for many years studied people's behaviors.

The MBTI provides a measure of personality by looking at eight personality preferences that all people use at different times. These eight preferences are organized into four bipolar scales. When you take the test, the four preferences that you identify as most like you (one from each scale) are combined into what is called a type.

The Four Scales Measured by MBTI

Scale	Refers to	Key Activity
Extroversion (E)/ Introversion (I)	How a person is energized	Energizing
Sensing (S)/ Intuition (N)	What a person pays attention to	Attending
Thinking (T)/ Feeling (F)	How a person decides	Deciding
Judging (J)/ Perceiving (P)	Lifestyle a person adopts	Living

Your personality type is determined and represented by a specific combination of these preferences. Jung indentified the first three categories. Extroversion/introversion refers to whether you are energized by the external world around you (things, places, people), or by the inner world of reflection and contemplation. Sensing/intuiting refers to whether you gather information by collecting facts, data, things measured by the five senses, or through a patternlike, theoretical approach. Thinking/feeling refers to whether you make decisions in a logical, cause-and-effect objective way or in a subjective, relational, interpersonal, feeling-oriented way. Isabel Myers and Katherine Briggs added to Jung's three categories a fourth — judging/perceiving, which refers to how you prefer to act in the world, in a decided, ordered way (judging) or in a flexible, more spontaneous way (perceiving). Although people use all of the preferences at different times, their MBTI scores yield a four-letter type (e.g., ESTJ) that indicates the four preferences they prefer to use most often in gathering information and making decisions. The various combinations create sixteen different personality types, each with its own way of looking at the world, each with its own strengths and challenges.

The theory of psychological type can help people understand interpersonal communication, team effectiveness, and organizational dynamics. MBTI has been used as a tool by small businesses and large corporations, as well as government agencies and education institutions, to help people in organizations better understand themselves and their behaviors. IBM, Procter and Gamble, the U.S. Naval Academy, even the Roman Catholic Church have used MBTI. The Presbyterian Church published for its congregations a book inspired by MBTI and called it *The Sum of the Parts.* In its annual report, one company listed employees' types next to their names. For management, MBTI can help clarify how to restructure the company at the individual and organizational levels. Too often managers ignore the individual differences among people they select to work together; they're unaware that there may be a job you loathe that another personality type would die to get. Using MBTI to decipher the personalities of the players in a group, managers can match coworkers more appropriately, prompt individuals to communicate and solve problems more effectively, and therefore improve overall teamwork. Understanding your and other people's personality type will help you address and improve on your weaknesses, and will guide you to play to your and other people's strengths in romantic, family, and business relationships.

One of the most important things to remember about the MBTI measurement is that it does not measure good or bad, intelligent or stupid characteristics. Each type can have an extraordinarily high IQ.

Taking the Brain Type Institute Test

I first met Jonathan Niednagel almost a decade ago. He has the most uncanny and amazing ability to tell you who you are, what motivates you, and how you can best interact with other people. Jon speaks not of different psychological types but of different brain types. Today Jon is Director of the Brain Type Institute in California. Applying twenty-first-century technology to Carl Jung's psychological types, Jon has correlated specific brain regions to each of Jung's typological preferences and linked specific motor skill traits to each of the sixteen brain types. Jon's research also consists of evaluating each brain type by DNA analysis — he believes genetic testing will soon provide a scientific and measurable way for identifying the unique behavioral characteristics and differences in mankind. "I can travel around the world, to other countries and continents where I don't even speak the language, and I can tell people exactly who they are. People think I'm psychic. This has happened quite often. I knew that preferences had to have a genetic basis. We didn't have the technology to delve into that, but now we do." Now that technology is arriving. University of Iowa researchers report that PET scans showed differences between the brain activity of introverts and extroverts. Introverts have increased activity in the frontal lobes of the brain and anterior or front thalamus, which are associated with planning, remembering, and problem solving. Extroverts have increased activity in the anterior cingulate gyrus, temporal lobes, and posterior thalamus, which are are associated with tasks such as driving, listening, or watching. These observations suggested to the researchers that there is an underlying biological cause for differences in personality.

Jon has generously allowed us to include in this book his brain-type test, including directions, scoring, and interpretation. It is, in short form, the very best of the personality-type tests I have come across for the purposes of this book. I use it in my own family and with many people I work with.

Directions

In the following questions you must make one of two choices: a or b. You will find that a third choice, c, is provided as well. It wants to know if the person who knows you best (spouse, relative, friend, and so forth) would disagree with your answer. If you feel he or she would disagree, then check c, too. Therefore, on certain questions you may have two answers checked, either a and c, or b and c.

The questions are not meant to be difficult. Set aside some time for yourself without interruptions. Perhaps, in some cases, you will feel like choosing both a and b. Even if you agree with both answers, check the one with which you agree more.

To yield an accurate description of yourself, it is imperative that you answer the questionnaire honestly. Answer as you really are, not as the person you would like to be.

As much as possible, try to make choices outside the context of your job. In other words, questionnaire results can be altered if you interpret too many questions with your job in mind. The fact that we all have certain job responsibilities and strong interests should not be used to cloud the results. Therefore, try to think of situations in which you are most free to be yourself.

Again, there are no right or wrong answers. Once you have completed the survey, you will be on your way to making some exciting discoveries.

The Brain Type Institute Survey

Answer on each of the following 20 groupings of phrases and word pairs, which choices most accurately describe you. Record your answers in the columns following the questionnaire.

1. a. higher energy level, sociable
   b. lower energy level, reserved, soft-spoken
   c. close associate probably disagrees

2. a. interpret matters literally, rely on common sense
   b. look for meaning and possibilities, rely on foresight
   c. close associate probably disagrees

3. a. logical, thinking, questioning
   b. empathetic, feeling, accommodating
   c. close associate probably disagrees

4. a. organized, orderly
   b. flexible, adaptable
   c. close associate probably disagrees

5. a. outgoing, make things happen
   b. shy, do fewer things
   c. close associate probably disagrees

6. a. practical, realistic, experiential
   b. imaginative, innovative, theoretical
   c. close associate probably disagrees

7. a. candid, straightforward, frank
   b. tactful, kind, encouraging
   c. close associate probably disagrees

8. a. plan, schedule
   b. unplanned, spontaneous
   c. close associate probably disagrees

9. a. seek many tasks, public activities, interaction with others
   b. seek more private, solitary activities with quiet to concentrate
   c. close associate probably disagrees

10. a. standard, usual, conventional
   b. different, novel, unique
   c. close associate probably disagrees

11. a. firm, tend to criticize, hold the line
   b. gentle, tend to appreciate, conciliate
   c. close associate probably disagrees

12. a. regulated, structured
   b. easygoing, "live and let live"
   c. close associate probably disagrees

13. a. external, communicative, express yourself
   b. internal, reticent, hold things in
   c. close associate probably disagrees

14. a. consider immediate issues, focus on the here-and-now
   b. look to future, global perspective, "big picture"
   c. close associate probably disagrees

15. a. tough-minded, just

    b. tenderhearted, merciful

    c. close associate probably disagrees

16. a. preparation, work-minded

    b. go with the flow, play-minded

    c. close associate probably disagrees

17. a. active, initiate

    b. reflective, deliberate

    c. close associate probably disagrees

18. a. facts, things, seeing "what is"

    b. ideas, dreams, seeing "what could be," philosophical

    c. close associate probably disagrees

19. a. matter-of-fact, issue-oriented, principled

    b. sensitive, people-oriented, compassionate

    c. close associate probably disagrees

20. a. control, govern

    b. latitude, freedom

    c. close associate probably disagrees

	I				II				III				IV		
	a	b	c		a	b	c		a	b	c		a	b	c
1				2				3				4			
5				6				7				8			
9				10				11				12			
13				14				15				16			
17				18				19				20			
	E	I			S	N			T	F			J	P	

How to score your test

To find your Type profile, add the number of a, b, and c responses in each column. (There are four columns and eight numbers in each column.) In column 1, simply total the number of checks of a, b, and c in the boxes below. This shows your E (extroversion) versus I (introversion) score. Add the results of columns 2, 3, and 4 as you did in column 1. This shows your S (sensation) versus N (intuition) score, T (thinking) versus F (feeling) score, and J (judging) versus P (perceiving) score.

Next, circle the one letter of each pair that is the highest number. Your Type is now expressed as a four-letter combination.

WHAT ABOUT THE "C" RESPONSES?

The number of c responses you find will tell you two things. First, it will serve as a tiebreaker if your a and b responses are equal. Second, it will tell you to use caution in evaluating your own preferences. For example, if you checked three J responses, two P responses, and three c responses, you will have to take some additional time considering your true preferences. You will have to pay special attention to the responses the c's were opposing. For example, if all your J choices also have c's marked, you evidently think someone who knows you well would consider you a P. Your score would actually differ if your friend's c responses were tallied. As you can see, the c responses serve as a warning that your self-perception may not agree with the way others see you.

SO WHAT'S YOUR TYPE?

Now that you've taken the questionnaire, you're probably anxious to know the meaning of the results. You have a combination of four letters that describes your typological design, one that is different from fifteen other types. For a brief description of your type, see the summary chart of the sixteen types in the workbook. There you may read about your own type and see how it compares to others. The profiles were developed for this book by Jon Niednagel. Jon spent a great deal of time, thought, and effort to get each of these just right. For each type you'll first find an overview, then popular career choices. The section on popular career choices will give you a sense of whether what you're doing is a true fit to your personality type. Mostly, it can give you a sense of reassurance. For instance, if you are a "wordsmith" and want to write the great American novel but feel pressured to run for office or start a new company . . . don't! Aside from this reassurance, don't feel you should abandon something you love because you don't have exactly the right fit. For instance, former Apple Computer President John Scully long said he wasn't an administrator but was more of a thinker and imagineer. At the top, you can always place a team around you to do what you can't or don't want to do! The section "what is important to know" about each type will give you a sense of how to approach different personality types. First, look at their inherent skills, the things you should value them for. Second, be sure they are happy doing what they do. Third, consider their common job descriptions. If you practice emotional broadcasting suggested in the Step that follows, the entry "Best approach to this personality type" in the workbook will give you a sense of who your audience is, so that you can correctly target your approach. Finally, you'll find examples of people who may share your personality profile.

Keep in mind this is only a brief description, not a summary of your whole personality. After you've studied your profile, return to read the rest of the chapter.

How to use what you've learned

To find out whom you're dealing with, give people the test! Reveal your own personality type and discuss how understanding your differences and shared strengths can better help you work together. For instance, I found "investigator" types always miffed at the big picture because they were concentrating so hard on the fine details of actually investigating. The compromise I now strike with "investigators" is that I help them nail down those details, but have them understand why I value the big picture, perhaps as a framework within which to place the hard facts. Give 50 percent of your message based on who the other person is. For example, if you're talking with an introvert, you want to ask questions, give him or her time and patience. It's OK for you to be you and to express what's on your mind based on who you are, but you will not be as effective as when you direct 50 percent of the message based on who the other person is. You have to realize that personality type is inborn wiring, and you won't be able to change your or the other person's type, much as you may want to. The way to change is to take practical, simple, realistic, measurable steps, and the very first step is understanding your and the other person's brain type. As you look around you, start noticing how different types operate; and then custom-tailor your communications.

You may not agree with everything (or anything!) that is written about you, but if you have answered the questionnaire true to yourself, the majority of traits and habits will be accurate. If you really have a struggle with the description of your personality, it is likely that you didn't answer all questions in accordance with your true self, and one or more of your preferences are wrong. If this is the case, don't be concerned. Accuracy cannot be guaranteed by a questionnaire. It is only the first step in discovering your inherent characteristics. If your answers are equivocal, you may want to take the MBTI test. Professional psychologists can administer the MBTI test. You can also find an excellent test in David Keirsey's classic book *Please Understand Me.*

Now that you've had a chance to examine your personality type, here are a few other points.

Work on your strengths: Everyone has strong and weak points. You have two options: Either work on your strong points, or try to neutralize your limitations. Yuri Hanin, Ph.D., of the Research Institute for Olympic Sports in Finland, says, "Only by developing your strong points will you enter the level of excellence. You have to think, 'What are my strong points and how can I further develop them?' It's not helpful or worth it to work on your limitations. 'Weak points' — we don't even use that vocabulary here."

Strengthen your weaknesses: Despite Yuri's advice, the goal is to develop a balance. So, if you're a strong judger, it's important to develop some sense of being a perceiver to be more measured. Explore areas outside your type. People who are the most persuasive and most successful are those who are willing to work on areas they're not strong in. For example, if you're an introvert and you know that introverts are sometimes shy or that introverts make you feel like you have to reach out to them whereas extroverts reach out to you, you might try behaving more like an extrovert.

Don't take strengths to the extreme: We tend to take preferences too far; and a strength taken too far can become our greatest weakness. We're so comfortable with what we are that our behavior comes automatically. For instance judgers can quickly become too controlling. I'm always impressed by bosses who are control freaks but are willing to give it up to let others live. It's even more important for parents who are control freaks to understand that although control comes easily to them, they should "ease up" because they're crushing their children.

Learn more: Taking a questionnaire is only one step in the process to determine your true brain type. The Brain Type Institute offers other and more reliable helps, such as CD-ROMs, video tapes, and personal evaluations. Consider your questionnaire results with objectivity and caution.

Of course, personality testing is a simplification, but it is useful. Think about how you've behaved in the past. How have you handled people's different styles? Have you aggressively attacked by saying, "You must change! Stop it. Don't do this, don't do that!" The result of your efforts? People end up feeling worthless, guilty, and the problem itself is exacerbated; you have engaged in what Stephen Montgomery calls "The Pygmalion Project," an attempt to transform your loved ones into what you want them to be. The entire Pygmalion Project is itself destructive and futile, and you should substitute for it an understanding of types. Understanding brain types will help you understand your family, friends, and coworkers. By talking with people you'll start to get a sense of their psychological type. Even two-year-old children clearly express their preferences.

If you want to be happy and motivated, if you want to maximize your potential and consistently be "in the zone," you have to know your brain type and try to understand other people's brain types. Remember the number one rule for success is that you operate within your biological makeup. If you're aiming for long-term fulfillment and joy, then you will want to pursue vocations and areas of interest that fit your inborn makeup. When you interact with others, channel your positive thought in a direction that suits the other person's typology. Remember, however, that, like two sets of fingerprints, no two people are exactly alike. Play to your strength and play to the other person's strength . . . in order to succeed. In the following Step we'll look more closely at emotional broadcasting and how to approach people whose personality types are different from yours.

Step 4: Practice
Emotional Broadcasting

It's 10:37 A.M. on a beautiful Monday morning and you're on top of the world. But as you walk past the boss's office, you catch a glimpse of the old man. He's not happy. He glances briefly in your direction. Was that a scowl? Was he looking past you or directly at you? You quickly review the last six months. Are you the source of his unhappiness? Were you less productive than you should be? Was it something *you* did wrong? Should you get your résumé ready? Chances are his mood has nothing to do with you. But that still doesn't change the precipitous drop in your own mood. And you're not alone. Look around the rest of the office. Angry, depressed, glum, and moody bosses transmit their moods to others around them. Although not a word was spoken, emotional changes took place in those who came into contact with the boss. Stephen Schwarzman, the President of the highly successful Blackstone Group, told me he carefully guards himself not to express an untoward emotion, so that if he's having a rare bad day, half his office isn't looking elsewhere for work. John D. Rockefeller in his day was also very guarded about revealing negative emotions around any people he worked with. And it's not just the boss. "Anxiety is contagious" is a saying in psychiatry. Sit with someone who is nervous and testy and fidgety and soon you'll feel the same. Spend some time with someone really down in the dumps and chances are you'll soon be along for the ride. But take a friend or colleague in an absolute state of bliss or real inner peace, there is a powerful emotional carryover to all those around him.

CONVENTIONAL WISDOM: Wear your feelings on your sleeve.

THE BIOLOGY OF SUCCESS: Broadcast winning emotions to build a winning team around you.

The heart of emotional broadcasting is this: it's not what you say but the emotional changes you effect in those around you that count. You may overhear a conversation filled with seemingly meaningless grunts, "yups," "uh hunhs," and "hmmms," only to discover that the exchange is imparting and reinforcing a highly positive mood transfer. Mood is infectious. Unfortunately, too few of us consciously make a planned effort to infect those around us with an emotion that brings them or us closer to success. There are countless superbright people who just throw the facts out in conversations or presentations but make no impact at all . . . for example, presidents of some high-tech companies. That may explain, in part, the utter lack of loyalty some employees have to their Silicon Valley start-up firms.

Michelangelo, the Renaissance sculptor, painter, architect, and poet, believed that the artist did not *invent* but only *liberated* a statue from a block of marble or stone. In other words, the statue, for example an angel, already existed as a potentiality in the block, and the artist just uncovered it.* In the same way, look at the people around you as beautiful designs to liberate with the power of your emotional broadcasting. You may get the impression that emotional intelligence is inborn, like a traditional IQ, and only those born with facile emotional communications can practice it. The more likely problem is that many of us are reticent to share our emotions or just plain don't know how to.

Let's face it, many of us in America were never trained to use our emotions. We're emotional stone walls. Even worse, when emotions come at us, we're queasy and uncomfortable. Sure we have professional executive emotions — anger, anxiety, low mood — but we have difficulty expressing positive emotions such as joy, happiness, or even love. So to begin with, try to experience uplifting emotions. That can be as simple as seeing a great movie, going to a great church service or inspirational speech, or listening to an opera or a symphony. Once you begin to experience uplifting emotion, you'll be less inhibited about expressing emotion. Sure it's awkward

---

*See Anthony Blunt, *Artistic Theory in Italy, 1450–1600* (Oxford: The Clarendon Press, 1956), pp. 73–74.

at the start. Dean Ornish realized in working with heart disease patients that expressing emotion was important. We had dinner several years ago and we were discussing emotions and I could feel how awkward the emotional connection was between us — as physicians, we weren't used to communicating on that level. Several years later, Dean has become the master of emotional broadcasting.

The Biology of Emotional Broadcasting

Emotion is at the fundamental core of motivation. Our entire emotional system is built to motivate and prioritize thinking, to energize behavior in order for us to act on what's important, reports Peter Salovey, Ph.D., Professor of Psychology at Yale University. People who have deficiency in emotional skills may have difficulty focusing their behavior, thinking, and acting on what is most important at the moment; they may also have difficulty communicating their emotions to motivate others. If you're having a tough time finishing a project, think for a moment — what emotional energy do you have? If people aren't working with you, think about what kind of emotional support you are giving them. The best people I've worked with gave me an emotional charge. Emotion motivates, directs, and prioritizes what we do. Most of us relegate emotion to a secondary tier in terms of management, but remember, it is the fundamental way that the human brain prioritizes what it's going to do. So the next time you write down a list of priorities, try to associate strong positive emotions with them. Think of a great sales manager. She is primarily a great cheerleader, creating such positive emotion in the workforce, that they'll run through walls of fire to perform. That doesn't mean you have to be a boiling pot of emotion. Legendary Harvard crew coach Harry Parker rarely needed to say a word to his oarsmen. He relied instead on a taciturn emotional support, which most casual observers would have mistaken for a block of granite. But speak to members of his crews — they'd jump into a burning fire for a tiny glimmer of Harry's approval.

Professor Salovey was the first to coin the phrase "emotional intelligence." "Emotional intelligence is about how well you understand emotions, both your own and those of others," he says. Being emotionally intelligent means knowing how to regulate emotions, and using emotions as creative and complex tools to solve problems. Our traditional notions of what makes a person intelligent, what opens up the doors of life's success, are too narrow. Traditional IQ is overemphasized. Understanding emotions in oneself and in others is underemphasized. You can be a lot smarter and a lot more successful by opening up your mind to emotions and learning emotional broadcasting. Here's how.

Emotional Broadcasting: A Practical Guide

1. Put out

"Emotional broadcasting" means actively gathering your own emotions and carefully transmitting them to all the important people in your life to unlock an emotional response in them. When you make others feel better, they'll make you feel better. You are mobilizing energy. Which direction is the energy flowing? If you're constantly "wanting wanting wanting," you will be miserable. Remember teenage puppy love? You desperately wanted to be loved, but acted in so many goofy and strange ways that all you did was get hurt. But as soon as you were doing and caring for someone else you got energy and happiness in return . . . and better health. Positive feedback is a strong immune-system builder.

DON'T BE AFRAID TO SAY "I LIKE YOU"
Emotional broadcasting can be deceptively simple. Joe Gerard is in the *Guinness Book of World Records* as the best car salesman ever. He could consistently sell five cars and trucks a day every day he worked. One of the things he did was keep a list of all his customers (at one point, 20,000). Every month he would send them a greeting card. And although the outside of the card changed according to the season and occasion, the inside of the card never did; he would always write the same thing: "I like you." "Compliments, statements of affinity, statements of liking lead to positive reactions," says Robert Cialdini, Ph.D., Professor of Psychology at Arizona State

University and author of the classic *Influence: The Psychology of Persuasion.*

TRAIN YOUR EMOTIONS

I'll be the first to admit, it's really tough to put out. Sure, it's a great idea to broadcast you emotions, but many of us were taught not to wear our emotions on our sleeve. Many of us have become emotional recluses. And if you're the boss, it's even tougher. Why bother? So if you feel you can't, fake it and soon you'll feel it! Try to engage a performer's skills when you want to reset your mood. If you want to feel happy, act happy; if you want to feel optimistic, act optimistic. Disciplined acting and disciplined thinking are the same — two arms of changing emotions. What professional actors do is move their emotions at will. That's what experts at the training center LGE Performance Systems teach athletes — acting skills to move emotions in a certain direction. Athletes learn how to move their faces, shoulders, and other parts of their bodies in order to summon the right response. Emotion is the result of underlying physiology. What you feel is a cascade of neurological, physiological systems — anger, fear, and so on — and by performing emotionally, you can change your emotional set. When you need to feel a certain response, act out the response and you will find that you have summoned it. By using acting skills, you will actually be modulating the parts of your brain which control your emotional response.

Even if you feel that you can't do it, say to yourself, "Yes, I can; yes, I can." Affirmation can help change a belief system, so that you can perform in an area you thought you didn't like at a level you didn't think possible. Sports psychologist Jim Loehr says: "We put people through emotional workouts. We show them how better to modulate their emotions to produce their best. We help people build skill sets, or new habit responses, capacities that help someone change their feeling about something." Take Dan Jansen, the famous speed skater, as an example. He didn't like skating the 1000 meter. Jim trained him into wanting to skate the 1000; so every day Dan would say to himself "I love to run the 1000 meter," and then he won that race. He wrote a book about it, *Full Circle*. Belief systems lead to appropriate emotional responses and a great performance.

SHARE

When I was at CBS Evening News, one simple way we used to open up to one another was through share time. In the morning, our first fifteen minutes were devoted to what had happened to each of us in our private lives — fights, betrayals, scoldings, missed opportunities. We were honest to the point of becoming extremely entertaining. The routine was like stand-up comedy, and everyone came back for more. Since we weren't discussing work, there was no real risk, but it helped immeasurably in terms of bonding with each other. Sharing is a great way to start any good conversation. Surround yourself with people who make you happy, people with positive moods, and share with them.

ALLEVIATE GUILT

My ten-year-old once came home with a bad report card. He felt plenty guilty about it. In America, many of us trade on guilt for motivation. Instead, I said, "Look, you're smart, you're a good student, why don't we work together for better grades?" Both at work and at home, a positive message is infinitely more powerful than guilt. There is a connection between helping and alleviating guilt. Since you know the guilt is there, you needn't trade on it. You'll gain unending gratitude by rewarding with understanding rather than reproach.

DON'T BE AFRAID TO SAY HOW YOU CAN HELP

Virgil said, "Follow an expert." We all like experts. One of the things some of the brightest people most often fail to do is to inform others that they are experts. Though announcing your expertise may seem boastful, it is effective, says Professor Cialdini. People want to know what the experts think. Demonstrate your competence, standing, and status. If you have credentials, experience, awards, background in a particular arena, show or tell people. A hospital with problems getting stroke patients to do their exercises found that patients started to comply once they saw on the wall the physical therapists' diplomas certifying the therapists as experts. One of the best ways to build an emotional bond is to let the person know that you are there ready, willing, and *able* to help. Just the offer is often an icebreaker. Be generous. Don't wait for other people to broadcast willingness; beat them to the punch. It will be worth it.

2. Avoid the "Pygmalion Project"

Do you find personality traits in your spouse, coworkers, employees, even in yourself that you just can't stand? Does it get in the way of what you want most in life? Have you ever left a social gathering knowing you had really made an impression, only to find that your spouse had a list of things you shouldn't have said? Are you having trouble with those around you, wishing they would accept your constructive suggestions? Or are you on the receiving end of those suggestions and having a hard time accepting criticism? Do you feel you are not loved or appreciated for who you are, only for what you accomplish for the team, organization, or family? If you've ever felt that way, it's not because you're just having a bad day. There's truth to your dislike and difference. As we've learned in the previous Step, "Play to Your Strengths," psychologists confirm that people of different psychological types can very well have a hard time working together because each has a distinctive way of perceiving the world and making decisions. While men may be from Mars and women from Venus, if your boss is from Pluto, your secretary from Mercury, and your kids from Jupiter, you're going to have a very rough go!

How do you handle it? Remember how Henry Higgins in *My Fair Lady* tried to undertake a total remake of Eliza Doolittle. Those of us who try to remake those around us suffer from wanting to implement what author Stephen Montgomery calls the "Pygmalion Project." And since our differences are hard-wired, all such attempts at changing or remaking others will fail. Remember what Jonathan Niednagel of the Brain Type Institute said: "Typological and genetic research now concur that certain aspects of our personality are paramount and unchangeable." So stop trying to change people and start trying to understand them. Try to assess what the personality types are of those around you. Ask colleagues, friends, business associates, and family to take the test in "Step 3: Play to Your Strengths"! Then turn to the workbook section for the chapter "Play to Your Strengths" and review how best to approach their personality type. Live and let live to get the job done. Understand how you should approach different personality types, and then start emotional broadcasting.

3. If you can't say anything good . . .

. . . Don't say anything at all. In terms of emotional broadcasting, if you don't have anything good to say, if you're not in a positive mood, don't go "on the air." This realization has changed the way I live. If I'm in a foul or low mood, I try to avoid people. If I'm really upset about something someone has done, I don't go after them, but try to hold it in until I can deliver a more positive message. If you really have to vent, don't direct your negative emotions at someone, just share with them why you're in such a foul mood so that they don't feel that they're being attacked. To broadcast positive emotion you need positive mental energy, which is why the measures in Part One of this book are so crucial to engendering positive emotions.

4. Create a "neural network"

Scientist long ago found that a single computer could only do so much, no matter how much memory was added, no matter how powerful the chip, no matter how fast the data pathways. However, if they tied many computers together, immense power resulted. The best example of all is the internet, whose power derives from the number and variety and uniqueness of the connections. No matter how smart you are, no matter how hard you work, no matter how strong your drive, there is a limit to what a single human mind can accomplish. I'll be the first to admit that for years I thought I could do it all alone, that pure drive and determination could accomplish anything. And then I discovered the enormous, amazing power of becoming part of a team. I call a team a "neural network," by which

I mean that you are tying your brain's processing power together with the brains of others on your team. The "neural network" has unleashed for me a sense of power and satisfaction such as I had never experienced before.

The purpose of emotional broadcasting is to transmit positive emotions to others in order to motivate them to work with you. I think of emotional broadcasting as reaching into other people's brains and directing their attention to what you'd like to accomplish together. In turn, as they give you emotional feedback, you are energized and motivated. This is called a positive feedback loop. You pour emotional energy into others and they, in turn, send it back to you. If you make a big enough effort to charge emotionally all of those who work with you, you can construct your own neural network. A now deceased friend of mine named Bob Stone created a huge national network around himself so he could gain emotional support in his struggle against cancer. This network of "Buffaloes," as he called them, has become one of the most fabled cancer support groups, giving emotional support to thousands of desperate patients and their families. Bob in turn outlived all predictions scientists made about his survival.

The neural network makes sense. Remember, many of the roughest computing problems are no longer handled by a large supercomputer, but by hundreds of computers linked together in a network to achieve tremendous processing power. The same can be true for human beings. The larger the neural network of friends and colleagues you create, the greater your own motivation and chance of eventual success. Think again of the amazing financial and informational power of the internet; the power derives from the sheer numbers of people the internet connects. When the first fax machine came out, it had no value. However, with each added machine, the growing network gained in value. Look at patients who recover; by grasping at the emotions of nurses, doctors, technicians, they build tremendous emotional support around them. Then look at a failed boss renowned for being tough and angry. When he's fired, there are no tears.

If emotional broadcasting sounds foreign and you and your colleagues at work can't approach this level of connection, ask yourself, "What's the dominant emotion I broadcast?" For many of us, it's nothing, a sterile emotional blank slate. For others, it's anxiety, fear, aggression, or even anger. Pledge to develop and use your emotions to benefit yourself, your family, and those around you.

Emotional support is extremely important for everyone and makes a difference in how well people can deal with traumatic situations. One of the things that makes relationships worthwhile is the quality of emotional support we receive from someone; if we don't get the emotional support we need, we look elsewhere. Emotional support is an important characteristic for selecting friends, coworkers, and spouses . . . but be careful how you do it! Be aware of your verbal strategy. There are strategies that make people feel better and verbal strategies that make people feel worse. Saying, for example, "It's okay that your boyfriend left you — he was a real weirdo-freak, and you deserve better" might seem to be a good affirming thing to say, but in fact it's insulting because it questions the judgment of a person who would go out with a "weirdo-freak" in the first place. Contrast that with comforting strategies, such as "You must be upset by this. You were together for so long. . . . Tell me what happened." Comforting strategies encourage people to articulate their feelings. Practice being aware of your feelings and the feelings of others. One way is to play "Act Me Out," a role-playing emotional practice game. Find someone you know and trust and tell them "You play me and I'll play you." Spend five minutes seeing if you can understand what it feels like to be that person.

5. Give up control

A big deal is going down the tubes. You scream for help, criticize your team for failing you, complain about lack of corporate support. Are you going to save the deal? No chance. Most of us have an idea of what a prototypical boss is: a super control freak who yells and screams and blames others. We hear over and over about mean bosses as the model for successful management. They practice what is called external control psychology. Remember New York's famous Queen of Mean, Leona Helmsley. She was famed for external control psychology and no one shed a tear when she went off to prison for tax evasion, yet many of us put external control psychology into action when we're having problems.

Monitor your own conversations and those you work with for destructive external control words — that is, words that criticize, blame, complain, threaten, and punish. Be wary of offering a reward in return for control, e.g., "If you go to bed, I'll give you an apple," as described in Alfie Kohn's book *Punished by Rewards*. "External control psychology destroys relationship because all humans are internally motivated, and genetically we will resist external motivation," says Dr. William Glasser, M.D., founder and president of the William Glasser Institute in California. External control psychology causes dysfunctional relationships, divorce, and failed careers. Many of us practice external control psychology. Even worse, we think that's what we're *supposed* to do, that we should punish and cajole in order to motivate. So what's the alternative? Dr. Glasser has come up with an excellent one: choice theory.

6. Give choice a chance

Choice theory says that we are internally motivated, not directed by red-faced, screaming, out-of-control bosses. Dr. Glasser describes choice theory in books such as *Choice Theory: A New Psychology of Personal Freedom* and *The Language of Choice Theory*. We are motivated by five basic needs, Dr. Glasser says:

1. Survival
2. Love, belonging, and connection
3. The need for power
4. Freedom from control of other people
5. Fun

Effective communication — whether through vocabulary or body language — often appeals to one of these five needs. Great communicators — whether Ronald Reagan, Bill Clinton, Walter Cronkite, or Winston Churchill — all project the promise that "if you listen to me, stick with me, you'll better satisfy one or more of your five needs." Winston Churchill promised England survival . . . and they got it.

Choice is also a matter of good health. Many bosses, accurately enough, say they don't get ulcers, they give them. But what about the poor soul who is on the receiving end? Those who feel the very most stress often have the very least control.

How do you give choice a chance? Start by eliminating external control words from your vocabulary when asking people to cooperate with you. You'll get people closer to you by explaining what you yourself can do. When addressing a problem, for example, tell the person what you can contribute, and then ask "What can you do?" "I call it 'The Solving Circle,'" Dr. Glasser counsels. "Instead of attacking, you say 'This is what I'll do to solve the problem; what can you do?' Once you learn choice theory, every time you make a choice with another human being, you choose to be closer. Always do something that brings you closer; never choose to be further away."

I work at NBC News, a division of General Electric, considered one of the best companies in the world. As a physician, I came from several work environments where creative tension was more the rule. Yet at NBC I have never heard an unkind word, never heard anyone scream or yell, blame or criticize. I've got to admit it was a pretty hard transition for me. You almost *had* to be nice. At bad times, like many people in our industry, I'd criticize, blame, or complain. Slowly I made the transition . . . and what a difference it has made. By offering encouragement and having the guts to give up external control psychology, I found the stories we all participated in as a team were far better than ones I could ever have done on my own. And NBC isn't alone. Ten years ago when the Chrysler corporation was concerned about morale on its assembly line, company management tried something radical. It gave the workers more control, and as a result the workers became more motivated, explains Michael Lewis, Ph.D., a psychologist at Rutgers University. Workers helped redesign a plant in St. Louis. The majority of employees said this made the difference between a happy work environment and an unhappy one. Now that they have more control over their lives, they feel happier.

ENTER SOMEONE'S "QUALITY WORLD"

Cooperation works best when you're in someone's "quality world" and they're in yours. "The Quality World," based on William Edwards Deming's work, assumes that we each have in our heads things, places, or people we have enjoyed and significant pleasures associated with these things, places, or people. If a teacher can get into a child's quality world, then the child will try to do his or her best in that teacher's class. You are your "quality world's" own gate-keeper. If someone repeatedly treats you badly, you will remove him from your quality world. When you remove people from your quality world, they basically cease to exist for you; they become a non-entity. But if you lose someone from your quality world, when a loved one dies, for example, it's a terrible thing; it's a great loss. Since our quality world is at the core of our lives, it is also a key concept in choice theory. You can't force yourself into someone's quality world; brainwashing does not work, but good communication might.

One of the most effective methods of giving ourselves a chance to enter someone's quality world is through a simple conversation. What many people miss is that in a conversation we communicate much more than simple information. You are first and foremost communicating mood. I'm a big believer in "bond first, deal later." Think of even the simplest negotiation. You're on an airline and would like your seatmate to lower the window shade. Obviously there's a reason you want the shade lowered — the light bothers you, you'd like to sleep or watch the movie. But this simple request may be resented or even rebuffed by your seatmate. If, however, once you got on the plane, you established an emotional "I like you" connection, your seatmate will likely gladly do you the favor. Why don't we do this? Too many of us begin our emotional conversations in the middle. That is, we've started the conversation in our heads, and fully expect that our listener has heard and understood every word. What's more, we've actually worked ourselves up emotionally so that the first emotion we emit is anxiety or even hostility.

I had had great difficulty communicating with my own sons, always trying to bring them into my quality world of classical music, competitive sports, and world politics. Only by giving that up and entering into their world of video games, toy stores, action figures, and Saturday morning cartoons, did I "get it." I walked into the den and saw my ten-year-old bonding with my younger brother. They were watching a baseball game together, talking about what a power hitter was. I'd always made the mistake of grabbing my kids kicking and dragging into my world rather than just relaxing and drifting into theirs.

7. Put positive emotions on display: smile

Pay close attention to your emotional displays. Remember that smiles, frowns, and all facial expressions communicate information. We're wired to respond to emotional displays, such as facial expressions, body posture, or tone of voice, all of which tell us whether we're safe or not.

So smile. Researchers say that smiling also helps you live a longer, happier life. Even if you are not happy, fake it. Experiments show that when people fake smiles, they actually do start feeling better. If you're having trouble faking it, remember that creating positive emotions increases activity of the zygomatic muscles (the smiling muscles), as shown on an electronic muscle activation test called an EMG. Negative emotion increases the muscle activity of the corregator muscle, the muscle of frowning and startle responses.

8. Surround yourself with success

Ever notice how fired up you get even going to a winning team's baseball game? Many of us experience vicarious success. A whole city may seem to do better when the home team is having a winning season. In a strong bull market, a whole city such as New York may suddenly feel successful. Success comes from successful environments. The same is true for corporations. General Electric breeds more successful managers than any place on earth. Successful families breed successful children. Look at Leopold Mozart's son Wolfgang Amadeus, the Adams family from Massachusetts, the Gates family — the children in these families vicariously experienced success around them and so awakened to the possibility of success. If you are in a dynamic company, school, or family, you'll experience and see success. If you're not, you need to place yourself in situations in which you can experience and feel success.

Real Broadcasting

During all of my years in television journalism, I have noticed again and again that emotional broadcasting does work; you really can emotionally cue another person . . . over the airwaves. In radio and TV broadcasting, listeners and viewers have the opportunity of tuning you out. They are looking for a certain style and content. You may find that you are being tuned out even if you have a highly charged emotional pitch. You need to be aware that different people collect information differently and that you may have to appeal to each of them at a different level. Many national news anchors are ENTJs, emoting thinking rather than feeling, and it works for them because the nature of their business is *not* to be nice! Viewers do want the facts and don't want to feel manipulated emotionally. But this factual approach leads to low likability scores. Exceptions such as Katie Couric and Oprah Winfrey went to the top of the profession because of their skills *and* their ability to connect emotionally with the audience.

In our professional and family lives we all have a chance to be remembered as terrific human beings. However, the likelihood of creating these fond memories will be greatly increased by the emotional ties we make today.

Step 5: Look to the Hereafter

⫴

The Power of Positive Thinking, by Norman Vicent Peale, was written nearly fifty years ago and has sold over five million copies. It is still in print today. What I find remarkable about Peale's book is that it championed the healing powers of prayer decades before science confirmed Peale's observations. Modern-day cynics might disregard prayer and speak scornfully of religion. But first-rate science has now demonstrated the amazing power of spirituality in general and prayer in specific. I don't mean to suggest that spirituality, religion, and prayer be adopted simply as another technique for improving mood and enhancing positive thought. The religious or spiritual impulse must first come out of deeply held beliefs, which are beyond the scope of this book. But if you have this impulse, then practicing your religious or spiritual belief will be extremely beneficial to your life.

> **CONVENTIONAL WISDOM:** Religion is for the weak and old.
>
> **THE BIOLOGY OF SUCCESS:** Get on your knees to succeed!

The Biology of Prayer

Scientific, not anecdotal, studies now show that prayer works wonders on health. Of the three hundred studies on spirituality in scientific journals, the National Institute of Health Research found that 75 percent showed that religion and prayer have a positive effect on health. I'm also recommending that you use spirituality to build positive thought and a great mental attitude. Consider the following studies.

One of the first studies to address the issue of prayer and health was a controversial study by Dr. Randolph Byrd. Dr. Byrd explored the benefits of intercessory prayer or prayer for others. He reported on the "Positive Therapeutic Effects of Intercessory Prayer in a Coronary Care Unit." This ten-month double-blind study took place in a large county hospital in San Francisco. Half the subjects were prayed for and half were not; not only did the subjects not know whether they were being prayed for or not, but the people praying also did not know the patients for whom they were praying. The study found that the patients who were prayed for had fewer cases of congestive heart failure, less pneumonia, less need for antibiotics, and fewer cardiac arrests than those who weren't. Although some scientists questioned Byrd's method and claimed that one can't control intercessory prayer for the group not prayed for (after all, their families might be praying for them), Byrd's study became a landmark in that it opened an important question. And several subsequent studies showed concrete health benefits of prayer.

In a study of thirty female patients recovering from hip fractures, those who regarded God as a source of strength and comfort and who attended religious services were able to walk farther upon discharge and had lower rates of depression than those who had little faith.

One study by Harold G. Koenig, M.D., Director of Duke University's Center for the Study of Religion/Spirituality and Health, measured interleukin-6 blood levels in a church group. High levels of interleukin-6 usually indicate a lowering of immune function, and the church group members had lower interleukin-6 levels, indicating enhanced immune function.

In another study, Dr. Koenig discovered that religion-active older people tend to have lower blood pressure than those who are less active. "The likelihood of having a diastolic blood pressure of 90 or higher, the level most often associated with increased risk for strokes or heart attacks, was 40 percent lower among those who attended a religious service at least once a week and prayed or studied the Bible at least once a day, than among those who did so less often."* In yet another study with the elderly, Harold Koenig, M.D., and David Larson, M.D., found that people sixty and older who attended religious services at least once a week were 56 percent less likely to have been hospitalized in the previous year than those attending services less frequently.**

A Dartmouth Medical School study found that of 232 patients who underwent elective heart surgery, the very religious were three times more likely to recover than those who were not. The most consistent indicator of survival was the amount of strength or comfort the patients said they received from their religious faith. In fact, the more religious they described themselves, the greater the protective effect. Of 37 patients who described themselves as "deeply religious," none died. The researchers also found that the more socially active patients had higher survival rates. More time spent in religious activity correlated with more overall happiness and satisfaction.

So the more religious you are, the better for your emotional health. That seems contrary to the conventional wisdom. How many times have you heard friends complain about a strict religious upbringing and about how much it "screwed them up." And how many times have you heard experts argue that authoritarian religious upbringing or doctrine may damage mental health. New research indicates that the only damage done is when people abandon their religion. Listen to these results from a large, long-term University of Pennsylvania study.

Professor Martin Seligman considered nine major religions in the U.S.:

Fundamentalist: These groups interpret their religious texts quite literally and impose a lot of day-to-day regulation upon their

---

*H. G. Koenig, L. K. George, H. J. Cohen, J. C. Hays, D. G. Blazer, and D. B. Larson, "The Relationship between Religious Activities and Blood Pressure in Older Adults," *International Journal of Psychiatry in Medicine* 28 (February 1998): 189–213.
**H. G. Koenig and D. B. Larson, "Use of Hospital Services, Religious Attendance, and Religious Affiliation," *Southern Medical Journal* 91 (October 1998): 925–932.

followers. Professor Seligman looked at three religions that show heavy religious involvement and influence.

Calvinists

Muslims

Orthodox Jews

Moderates: Groups who no longer blindly accept the faith.

Catholics

Conservative Jews

Lutherans

Methodists

Liberals: Groups who encourage individuality, tolerance, and skepticism. The individuals are free to decide the extent to which they believe any religious dogma.

Reformed Jews

Unitarians

"We found that the more authoritarian religions produce more hope and optimism. The questionnaire and analysis of sermons and liturgy showed that fundamentalist individuals were significantly more optimistic and hopeful than moderates, who in turn were more optimistic and hopeful than liberal individuals. The more frequently people participated in fundamentalist religious activities, the less likely they were to report emotional distress," Professor Seligman says. "A causal model that takes into account religious influence in daily life and the effects of religious involvement, religious hope, and religious liturgy on explanatory style seems to account exhaustively for the effect of fundamentalism on optimism." Of course, the more religious people might have been more optimistic to start out, but religion only strengthened their optimism. And as we've seen in "Step 1: Be an Optimist," a positive explanatory style is incredibly potent, performing as well as drugs in the treatment of depression and obsessive-compulsive disorder.

Why Prayer

Patients, say the experts, respond to prayer because it offers hope, a way to cope, a sense of peace, and an overall sense of well-being. Prayer also works as a form of meditation, counteracting stressful thoughts while lowering heart rate and breathing, slowing brain waves, and relaxing muscles.

For some, prayer is a way of actively changing oneself from within. I interviewed Hasan Al Turabi, the head of the National Islamic Front in Sudan. He sees prayer as a means of personal communication with God, but also as a form of self-improvement. In fact he also says prayer grants your request because it changes you and how you interact with other people. Morning prayers allow you to plan your day. Midday prayers give you a running assessment of how things are going. Night prayers allow you to reflect on what you have done right and wrong and to think about how you might do better tomorrow.

Today 50 of the 130 medical schools in America are teaching courses on spirituality and medicine. And that number is growing every day.

David Larson, M.D., President of the National Institute for Healthcare Research, and adjunct Professor at the Department of Psychiatry at Duke Medical Center and Northwestern Medical School, says that spirituality can become of paramount importance in medicine in death and dying. Dr. Larson maintains that 70–75 percent of gravely sick people cope with God's help, and half of those become more religious as they deal with their illness. And in her work with dying patients, Christina Puchalski, M.D., Assistant Professor and Director of Clinical Research at the Center to Improve Care of the Dying at George Washington University School of Medicine, and Director of Education at the National Institute for Healthcare Research, has found that number to be even higher, at

80–85 percent. "Man is not destroyed by suffering. He is destroyed by suffering without meaning," wrote Victor Frankl, M.D., in his classic *Man's Search for Meaning;* and the sick, even more than the healthy, find meaning through spirituality. When thinking of death and dying, patients' stress and anxiety levels go up dramatically, and people with religious commitment have lower levels of death anxiety, more coping skills, and more social support from their congregations. Since one-third of a person's lifetime health care cost is spent in the last year of life, the health benefits of spirituality also lower health care cost.

"I don't think we should just be looking at prayer and religious commitment; we should also look at spirituality in the more general sense of the term," Dr. Larson says. By spirituality, Dr. Larson means your relationship to a transcendent that gives meaning and purpose to your life — this transcendent that is greater than you can be a divine being, God, or something else, such as nature, an energy force, or even art. "Spirituality seems to be helped by a structure," Dr. Larson says; in other words, if you are practicing your spirituality with others within a belief system (e.g., going to church or synagogue or mosque), you seem to be able to reap greater health benefits. "We should look first at spirituality, then at religious or spiritual commitment, and then at the role of prayer in spiritual or religious commitment."

Prayer is communication with a transcendent. This communication can take two forms: prayer as speaking to the transcendent; or meditation as contemplating or listening to the transcendent.

Guide to Prayer

Develop your own spiritual program

Although the choice of a specific faith is not a medical but a personal decision, several physicians now actually recommend that people incorporate spirituality in their lives. "I encourage a spiritual program consisting of a) prayer, b) reading of scripture, c) worship attendance, and d) involvement with a faith community," says

Dale A. Matthews, M.D., author of *The Faith Factor* and Associate Professor of Medicine at Georgetown University School of Medicine.

a) Prayer: Although I can't create a formula for you because details of prayer are individually based, try to pray every day.

b) Reading of scriptures: Whatever your faith, read some sacred scripture every day.

c) Worship attendance: If you have religious belief, attend a religious service at least once a week.

d) Involvement with a faith community: Become involved with a worship community; find a comfortable place. People in worship communities help and encourage one another through good and bad times.

Of course I am only suggesting that you undertake prayer and worship if you have a religious belief; if you don't, try using meditation by itself.

How to meditate

Studies show benefits of meditation and other relaxation response techniques for PMS, anxiety, depression, heart disease, high blood pressure, chronic pain, and headache. Herbert Benson, M.D., Associate Professor of Medicine at Harvard Medical School, and author of *The Relaxation Response, Beyond the Relaxation Response,* and *Timeless Healing,* teaches his patients how to elicit the relaxation response. The relaxation response is achieved through many techniques within the old Eastern and Western religious traditions of Christianity, Judaism, Buddhism, and Hinduism. Physicians throughout the country are now using the relaxation response in their treatment of patients. Reports Dr. Christina Puchalsky: "I've had particularly good results with headache patients. Especially patients with tension headaches due to stressful lives can achieve almost 100 percent management with meditation. Some of the patients with migraine headaches have also done well when they've used meditation in combination with prophylactic medicine." She offers the following guidelines for meditation:

1. Select a word that is spiritual to you (e.g., peace, love, light, one). If you're religious, choose a word from your religious tradition, for example "Christ" or "ohm" ("ohm" comes from the Hindu tradition). In Christianity, this practice is called "The Centering Prayer." Father Thomas Keating, Cistercian monk priest at St. Benedict's Monastery in Snowmass, Colorado, was one of the founders of both the "Centering Prayer Movement," which started around 1975, and "Contemplative Outreach," which is an organization designed to support those introduced to centering prayer. Centering prayer is largely based on *The Cloud of Unknowing,* written by an unknown English fourteenth-century spiritual father who, in teaching a contemplative kind of prayer to a disciple, said: "Choose a word, a simple word, a single-syllable word is best, like God or love, but choose a word that is meaningful to you."

2. Find a quiet place for yourself. Choose a comfortable chair and sit with good posture, back erect, feet uncrossed and firmly on the ground, and eyes closed. If you feel more comfortable on a cushion, sit crosslegged on a cushion but make sure you keep your back straight.

3. Breathe slowly and deeply, in and out, in and out. While you're exhaling or breathing out, utter either silently or loudly the chosen word. Continue doing this for the amount of time that you're meditating. Focus all of your attention on the word. When thoughts cross your mind, don't engage them or hold on to them; just let them go by bringing your attention back to your word.

4. At the end of your meditation time, slowly open your eyes.

When you first start to meditate, you'll notice that your mind is busy, that thoughts keep popping up. Don't worry, let them go, focus again on the word, and you'll find that your mind will gradually quieten. Don't be impatient. It takes time and practice to learn to still your mind. At first, practice for five minutes a day. Do not set an alarm, but keep a clock nearby so that you can see it if you open your eyes after one minute. Start with five minutes and build up to what Dr. Benson recommends based on his studies — twenty minutes twice a day.

Try meditating for a month and then decide how much you like it. Remember, people who can meditate for hours have been doing it for years. Father M. Basil Pennington, author of *Centering Prayer* and monk at St. Joseph's Abbey, an abbey of the Cistercian Order (also called the Trappists) in Spenser, Massachusetts, explains that St. Joseph's is a contemplative monastery in which one's whole life is geared to prayer. The monks awaken before 3:00 A.M. for individual prayer, then have community chants and readings, and then they have several more hours of contemplative prayer before starting to work at 8:00 A.M. The monks have several additional prayer sessions throughout the day and then end the day at 7:40 P.M. when they gather in church again for a final prayer service. At 8:00 P.M. they retire to their rooms where they often continue to pray! And the Trappists are not alone. Michael Wenger, Dean of Buddhist Studies at Zen Center in San Francisco, reports that monks at the center have several 30- to 40-minute meditations every day, an all-day meditation once a month, and, once or twice a year, a 5- to 7-day meditation in which the monks silently sit, walk, eat, and work in mindful meditation!

Says Father Thomas Keating: "Everyone needs an oasis of solitude and silence in this noisy and overactive society in which we live in the West. We need a daily period of being present to our deepest self in order to balance all the other things we do and to remain fully human."

Step 6: Create a Blueprint for Success

———— ||||||| ————

Remember the stories we told as children and teenagers? To create the illusion of success, we manufactured stories: I'm going to go to Harvard, I'm going to make the soccer team, I'm going to buy a Jaguar and take the prettiest girl or handsomest boy to the prom . . . even . . . I'm going to grow up and become president. We created a blueprint through imagination and inspiration. However, the greater satisfaction was actually living to tell the tale. Early in life we told short stories that spanned a few months or several years. We boasted to others about directions our careers might take. Now fast-forward to the end of life. Those who are the most satisfied, those who feel that their lives have been a crowning success, have a great story to tell. It needn't be a consistently happy story, but it does need to be a complete and fulfilling story.

What about stories makes them so important? Howard Gardner, Professor at the Harvard Graduate School of Education, writes: "Leaders achieve their effectiveness chiefly through the stories they relate."* Look at any great leader, and there is a story by which he or she leads. To lead our own lives in the direction of greatest success, we need to plan, direct, and live out the stories we have created.

CONVENTIONAL WISDOM: Titles count.
THE BIOLOGY OF SUCCESS: Create a life's story
    that breeds success.

—————

*Howard Gardner, *Leading Minds* (New York: Basic Books, 1995), p. 9.

Storytelling

Most Americans don't talk about a great success but a great success story. Most successes don't appear suddenly and fully formed; they bloom over years, even decades. The most essential part of our American culture is reflected in the expression "success *story*": Horatio Alger's rags to riches, an actress's discovery after years of obscurity, the great novelist winning the Nobel Prize late in life after years of political exile. We prize the story of the man or woman who arrived on our shores with nothing and rose to great riches or fame. However, the joy of their success isn't in hauling out a title or prize or bank account total, but in reveling in the journey.

I spent an evening with the late Trudy Elion, an extremely humble and dedicated biochemist. She told me her story of starting to work on Flag Day, 1944. She worked on nucleic acid metabolism. Although Watson and Crick's discovery of DNA was nearly a decade away, she still suspected DNA existed and had an important role in the growth of viruses. She found ways of using drugs to block DNA growth in viruses without harming the humans they infect. The result was the first truly effective and safe antiviral drug ever produced. The fallout from her work was enormous: antimalarial medications, anticancer medications, and the whole new field of antiviral drugs.* Never during her story did she mention that she had won the Nobel Prize! It was her journey, her work, and most of all her story that were most important. Sure, receiving the medal from the King of Sweden was a real thrill, but that's not the story that she used to tell.

The best success strategy is to imagine a story that you will want to live. So when someone says, "What do you do?" you have a story you're dying to tell. For a *Dateline* piece on pioneering heart surgery, I interviewed a woman who had eight children. She reveled in telling me about the dozen loads of laundry she'd do on Tuesday, about lugging home mountains of groceries. Her living room was a

---

*For an excellent discussion of Trudy Elion's achievements, see Tom Brokaw, *The Greatest Generation* (New York: Random House, 1998), pp. 303–306.

testament to her success, dozens of pictures of her children at every stage of life from diapers to wedding bells. She had even adopted a ninth child in her eagerness to have more children to raise. She had a total sense of satisfaction with her life. She wasn't a good mom, she was a tremendous mom. But you only get her sense of success by hearing the story, not the title . . . mother to nine.

Many of us don't take the time to construct in advance a "blueprint for success." Our story usually changes at each stage of life. When we're young, the story is how we got the new dollhouse or *Star Wars* set for our birthday. Then it's getting into a terrific college, then a great job. But it's only when you stop yourself long enough to really think about the *life* story you'd like to tell that you can pull together the focus and the motivation to achieve it.

Then you want to *live* your story. Think of the most famous and most satisfying and memorable movies: *Gone with the Wind, Titanic, The Lion King, Roots, It's a Wonderful Life.* They were epic tales of a life . . . satisfying stories. What's more, the protagonists in each movie embodied their story. That's also true of real-life leaders such as World War II and Marshall Plan architect General George Marshall. Howard Gardner writes of General Marshall: "Without necessarily relating their stories in so many words or in a string of selected symbols, leaders such as Marshall convey their stories by the kinds of lives they themselves lead and, through example, seek to inspire in their followers. . . . I argue that leaders exercise their influence in two principal, though contrasting, ways: through the stories or messages that they communicate, and through the traits that they embody."*

Finally, determine who your audience is. In high school your audience might have been the opposite sex. Even if you work in a large corporation, you need to have a story you can sell to fellow employees. Again in Professor Gardner's words, "even the most eloquent story is stillborn in the absence of an audience ready to hear it; even mediocre stories unimpressively related will achieve some

---

*Gardner, *Leading Minds*, pp. 37, 9–10.

effectiveness for an audience that is poised to respond."* But when thinking of your audience, take the long view. In the end, will you really care what your classmates or neighbors think? Is one-upmanship or keeping up with the Joneses really of any great importance? At some points life can be terribly confusing. For instance, your audience may not be ready — after all, history books are full of writers, composers, and visionaries who were only truly appreciated when they were long dead. Ultimately, you will want to impress the historians with the significance of what you have done. So even if you're truly a genius with superb sense for anticipating your greatness in the future, you might not find much of an audience in the here and now. That means your motivation must come from within.

In past centuries your audience would have been limited. Today, in the information age, you can reach millions of people in just a few seconds — and you can convince or deter in just a few moments. The difference between becoming an unsuccessful conspiracy theorist and an American president . . . is that many more people bought the president's story.

Find the Story within Yourself

In constructing your blueprint for success, look deep within yourself to uncover your unfulfilled needs. You have to identify your deepest, most important internal needs or deficiencies and then connect those to a life's story that will fulfill those needs. If there is only one question you ask yourself, it should be . . . what will my life's story be if I spend my life fulfilling that need? And then . . . is that story out of character for me? If your deepest needs are revenge or destruction, it's unlikely you'll feel great about living or retelling the story. Whatever your story, there is no substitute for plain hard work. Says William F. Buckley, "I know of no blueprint for success other than application."

---

*Gardner, *Leading Minds*, p. 291.

What if you're doing things you don't want in your story? That's the beauty of living your life by the story you'd like to become — if you're cheating, lying, or taking major diversions just to make money, and you don't want these actions in your story, then just don't do them. It wasn't just that the Monica Lewinsky scandal was wrong; it wasn't part of the story Bill Clinton wanted to tell. The next time temptation strikes, consider whether you want it in your obituary.

How to Live Your Story: The 10 Stages

1. Build motivation

Motivation is the engine that drives success. The ignition "must come from the inside," says sports psychologist James Loehr, Ed.D. The very best at anything "own" their motivation. When I was a U.S. ski team physician, there was only one distinguishing factor that characterized the Olympic medalists. They totally "owned" their motivation. Like many of us, their "also ran" teammates needed motivation from coaches, parents, boyfriends, or girlfriends. I remember most distinctly Bill Koch, who was both an Olympic silver medalist and a World Cup winner. He was the most inquisitive athlete I ever worked with, wanting to know the most detailed science of training. He didn't ask questions to impress, he asked them so he could own the material and use it to construct a world-class training program.

Many of us, myself included, read, write, create, train, and conduct parts of our professional lives out of a false sense of obligation . . . obligations to family or colleagues rather than to our deepest yearnings. Some of us work hard out of a spirit of revenge or keeping up with the Joneses. Only those with the strongest internal motivation develop the drive to be world class at whatever they do. The more passionate you are, the more the activity is going to fulfill strong internal motivations. Success feels best when it's fulfilling a deep-seated need. "Parents or coaches can help reinforce that ignition; mentors can help you overcome fear," says Jim Loehr. Surround yourself with people who are very motivated. Motivation is contagious. If you see people around you motivated, you get inspired. Also surround yourself with supportive, encouraging people. Even though ignition comes from the inside, you still need outside forces to reinforce that ignition.

Robert Singer, Ph.D, one of the most highly regarded sport psychologists, emphasizes the importance of finding a fulfilling activity. "You can only be self-actualized if you're undertaking an activity that you find personally fulfilling. Set goals that have to do with improving yourself. Of course, many times, both sources of motivation — internal and external — may operate. Many circumstances, for example poverty, create extrinsic motivation. The wishes to have power, fame, money, and recognition are all leading extrinsic motivation forces. But you always need to find pleasure and fulfillment to persist in an activity."

Since intrinsic motivation — that is, an internal system of beliefs — is so key to lifelong success, let's take a closer look at it. Intrinsic motivation is not just blind optimism. The energy of optimism has to be grounded in a basic belief that things will turn out well — for many people that is a belief in being able to improve oneself and one's situation, or the belief that the outcome of one's work will create a greater common good. Self-determination requires the active self-talk that optimists practice. Dr. Singer says, "High achievers in sports and elsewhere like to persist at achieving. They like the sense of fulfillment in doing well. You can develop that. Believe in yourself; believe that you can do it and do it consistently. You always have to be hungry. This has to do with your perception that you can do what needs to be done. Try to understand what it is possible for you to do . . . based on past experiences and an understanding of the present situation."

Linda S. Wilson, President Emerita of Radcliffe College, says: "We focused research on understanding positive outcomes, especially with regard to women's lives — we looked at men and women who've suffered awful problems, to find out what helped them overcome. Deep commitment and belief in what they were doing gave them strength; they had a resilience connected with their belief. If you don't have strong inner belief, obstacles will loom larger."

2. Create a vision

A word story of your life as you would like to have it unfold is not enough to succeed. That story must be transformed into a vision that inspires you to see your future the way it could be and should be. Many of us can only see our past paths, or the paths others have taken with their lives. We simply do more of the same. We get better and better at what we already do. But great vision projects boldly into the future. You should finally rise above all the mundane daily activities of living and working to see and *project* beyond the here and now into tomorrow; and that's far harder than it sounds. Take flight. Until the Wright brothers took the flight at Kitty Hawk or man walked on the moon, there was no past experience on which to base such visions, although there might have been the solid scientific principles in which to ground them.

Life's big winners see the situation as they envision it, then they *live* it. For two hours before the game, home run champ Mark McGwire visualizes how he'll play. Top performers, athletes, and executives alike, all create a visual plan of action. They can anticipate the anxiety, tension, pitfalls, and otherwise unexpected openings and breakthroughs that lie in the future. There are many excellent video- and audiotapes which will teach you how to visualize. I've found the easiest way to start visualizing is to lie down in the early evening after work and play some great music.

3. Create confidence

You have to believe in yourself and believe that you can perform and perform consistently. This has to do with your self-perception. Although the public sees success as a winning or loosing, the best success comes when people focus on performance goals rather than outcome goals. Remember what I said in the introduction to this book: Top performers don't say, "I want to be the number one in the world"; they say, "I want to try my best today." In sports as in life, many people determine self-worth by whether they win or lose, but that is unproductive. Many athletes don't do well in actual performance, because they're concentrating on trying to win instead of trying to do their best, and you could fall into the same trap. Define your self-worth according to improvement — work on improvement and measure your worth to yourself. Repeatedly ask yourself: "Am I performing at the level I should be, based on my experience of myself, and how could I improve myself?" Based on past experience and present situation, try to understand what it is possible for you to do. The most successful people I know in broadcasting focused on doing the best possible job in the present and shunned any notion of advancement . . . only to find themselves rising to the top. When they advance you, great managers are not looking at whether you are winning or loosing, they're looking at pure performance. Many of us perform as though we were in a lottery . . . we buy tickets and hope against hope to win. But the real joy and secret of winning is enjoying the performance.

4. Be bold

"Who dares wins" is the motto of the SAS, the Elite British Commando unit known as the Special Air Service. Those who win big have a real penchant for action. Many of us are afraid to stick out our necks . . . and with good reason. No one likes to get trashed, knocked down, or trounced. So be careful before you're bold. When you're really out there, you're exposed . . . so be sure you're right and you're ready for a good fight, that you have the allies and the ammunition you need — you can go it alone, but you won't have even a small fraction of the strength or resilience you'd have as part of a team. Once you've created your vision, surveyed the field, thoroughly prepared, built a team around you, and chosen your allies, go for it! Be bold. The greatest advances in all fields come as lightning strikes out of the blue — unexpected and contradictory to the conventional wisdom. Then stick to your guns. As long as you have a strong belief in what you do, you'll withstand the criticism, naysaying, and sometimes personal attacks of others. When you're bold, understand the difference between a Lone Ranger approach and a collaborative approach in leading. President Emerita Linda S. Wilson of Radcliffe champions the collaborative approach: "Collaborative styles often yield a more solid result. The more distributive approach has more staying power because ideas have been tested more and there's more opportunity, shared power, and deeper understanding; but this approach takes time . . . an up-front investment for long-term gain. The way the world works there is often not enough time for that, so there's a penchant for the Lone Ranger approach. A leader who can move with both the Lone Ranger and the collaborative approaches is best equipped to deal with the fast pace of change in today's world."

5. Explain your mistakes

High achievers have a highly rational and objective style of explaining themselves and their story. They have a specific reason for failure. Nothing saps motivation faster than the belief that you are beaten by forces that you cannot change. When something goes wrong, find the things that you *can* change. Say to yourself, "This is just a temporary setback, tomorrow I'm going to win again." Nearly 100 percent of the time, those who are tough, who keep coming back, *do* succeed.

6. Fight for integrity

Integrity is the single most important aspect of character. Dr. Michael DeBakey told me, "If you don't have integrity, you don't have anything. My parents made a clear decision as to what was right and wrong. Being honest is integrity. Children aren't born with responsibility. You have to teach them responsibility." Says Mark McCormack of integrity and a blueprint for success: "I think you should be extremely punctual, extremely dependable, very honest, and very hard working." Says Dr. John Silber, "There is only one aspect of success that is in the individual's power and that is moral and spiritual success. If you're born to caring parents and you're healthy, you can definitely live a moral life."

I'm a big believer in the continuous quality-improvement model. As you evolve, review all aspects of your work and personal relationships and assess your integrity. And when you're a crowning success, remember that integrity is even more important than ever before; without it, everything you've worked for can be tarnished or even destroyed. What's more, without integrity, you'll feel that once you've really made it, you somehow cheated and your victory will be that much more shallow for it. Tom Murphy was for years the Chairman of the ABC Television Network (Cap Cities/ABC) and is now Chairman of Save the Children: "A combination of energy and integrity are the most important for long-term success. Integrity means complete honesty, being a team player, not cutting people up. Energy comes from enjoying what you're doing."

7. Simplify your story

Construct a clear story. See the forest for the trees. Successful leaders are able to take very complex information and integrate it into a straightforward story they can sell to themselves and to others. Winston Churchill had a small audience for his story of German Doom in the early 1930s, but by the 1940s he was prime minister leading the campaign against the Nazis. Conversely, George Bush had a worldwide audience for his Gulf War campaign, but didn't have an economy story the American public would buy during the election two years later. Since in the end success is fulfilling deep inner needs, the first audience you want to satisfy is yourself; but after you've done that, make sure you can convincingly and clearly relate the story to others. Think, if you retold the story to your grandchildren, would they understand and applaud? Have you managed to weave perhaps a complicated and confusing plot into a clear and elegant story?

8. Embody your story

Remember Howard Gardner's words: "In addition to communicating stories, leaders embody those stories." We distrust politicians because they say one thing and yet their personal story embodies a contrary set of values. We reduce much of life's tension when we reconcile our stories with the way we live them.

9. Be eloquent

One trait of nearly all leaders is that they "are eloquent in voice, and many are eloquent in writing as well. They do not merely have a promising story; they can tell it persuasively," Professor Gardner writes.* The great thing about a life's story is that you own it. You can bring great eloquence as you add color, character, and boldness to the story of your life.

10. Be a hero or heroine

Honor and altruism are, I think, the two best qualities that a story can have.

I've had the privilege of chronicling the heroic deeds of doctors, relief workers, and the military over the last decade, during the genocide in Rwanda and Kosovo, the civil wars in the Congo, Sudan, Somalia, Kosovo, and Mozambique, and the Gulf War in Iraq and Kuwait. The satisfaction each of these heroes gained was from utterly abandoning his or her own self-interests while bravely coming to the aid of others. We all have ways of becoming heroes in our own life and of seeing our lives as a heroic adventure.

When I read the *New York Times* obituaries, I'm always struck by how so many of the most successful people are also biologically successful, living literally decades longer than the mean. Dr. Leonard Poon, Professor of Psychology at the University of Georgia, showed that there were common traits among people who lived to one hundred years or more. Many of those traits were the same ones that experts in the new field of the biology of happiness say makes a person happy: belief in God, volunteerism, activity in the community, ability to adapt to loss or change, supportive and connected relationships, an optimistic outlook, having a clear purpose in life . . . the same traits that underlie a biology of success. In the end, life is a dramatic and wonderful journey, during which we can grow and become vastly different and better people. If you think and plan carefully during that journey, living and embodying your story, you will achieve great success and great happiness.

---

*Gardner, *Leading Minds,* p. 34.

Workbook

Part One.
"Step 4: Eat for Mental Energy"

——— |||||||| ———

Below are tables for high-, moderate-, and low-glucose carbohydrates, maximum protein intake, lean proteins, and omega-3 fatty acids in fish. Read the charts in conjunction with the carbohydrate, protein, and fat sections of Step 4, "Eat for Mental Energy."

A.
HIGH-GLUCOSE CARBOHYDRATES

Food	Glucose Index	Food	Glucose Index
Hamburger bun	61	Pineapple	66
Ice cream	61	Angel food	67
Avon, canned	61	Croissant	67
New potato	62	Grapenuts (cereal)	67
Semolina	64	Puffed Wheat (cereal)	67
Shortbread	64	Breton wheat cracker	67
Raisins	64	Stoned Wheat Thins	67
Macaroni and cheese, boxed	64	Soft drink, Fanta	68
Beetroot	64	Maize, cornmeal	68
Flan	65	Mars Bar	68
Oat kernel	65	Crumpet	69
Rye flour	65	Wheat bread, gluten-free	69
Couscous	65	Shredded Wheat	69
High-fiber rye crispbread	65	Melba toast	70
Sucrose	65	Wheat biscuit	70
Cream of Wheat (cereal)	66	Potato, white, mashed	70
Life (cereal)	66	LifeSavers	70
Muesli (cereal)	66	Fruit, dried	70
Arrowroot	66	Golden Grahams (crackers)	71

HIGH-GLUCOSE CARBOHYDRATES (continued)

Food	Glucose Index	Food	Glucose Index
Millet	71	Puffed crispbread	81
Carrot	71	Rice Krispies (cereal)	82
Bagel, white	72	Rice cake	82
Water crackers	72	Corn Chex (cereal)	83
Watermelon	72	Potato, instant	83
Rutabaga	72	Corn Flakes (cereal)	84
Popcorn	72	Potato, baked	85
Kaiser rolls	73	Crispix (cereal)	87
Potato, boiled, mashed	73	Rice, instant	87
Corn chips	73	Rice, white, low amylose	88
Honey	73	Rice Chex (cereal)	89
Bread stuffing	74	Cactus jam	91
Cheerios (cereal)	74	Rice pasta, brown	92
French fries	75	French baguette	95
Pumpkin	75	Rockmelon	95
Donut	76	Parsnip	97
Waffle	76	Glucose tablets	102
Cocoa Puffs (cereal)	77	Maltose	105
Vanilla wafers	77	Tofu frozen dessert, nondairy	115
Broad beans	79		
Grapenut Flakes (cereal)	80	Table adapted with permission from the *American Journal of Clinical Nutrition* 62 (1995): 871–935.	
Jelly beans	80		

MODERATE-GLUCOSE CARBOHYDRATES

Food	Glucose Index	Food	Glucose Index
Capellini	45	Instant noodles	47
Macaroni, boiled 5 minutes	45	Bulgur	48
Romano beans	46	Baked beans	48
Linguine, thick durum	46	Green peas	48
Lactose	46	Corn, high amylose	49
Fruit loaf, wheat with dried fruit	47	Chocolate	49
		Rye kernel	50

MODERATE-GLUCOSE CARBOHYDRATES

Food	Glucose Index	Food	Glucose Index
Ice cream, low-fat	50	Sultanas	56
Tortellini, cheese	50	Pontiac, boiled	56
Yam	51	Potato, white	56
Kiwifruit	52	Pita, white	57
Banana	53	Orange juice	57
Pound sponge cake	54	Bran Chex (cereal)	58
Special K (cereal)	54	Peach, canned, heavy syrup	58
Buckwheat	54	Rice vermicelli	58
Sweet potato	54	Blueberry	59
Potato crisps	54	Pastry	59
Linseed rye	55	Rice, white, high amylose	59
Oatmeal	55	Digestive biscuits	59
Rich tea biscuit	55	Bran	60
Fruit cocktail, canned	55	Pizza, cheese	60
Mango	55		
Spaghetti, durum	55		
Sweet corn	55		

Table adapted with permission from the *American Journal of Clinical Nutrition* 62 (1995): 871–935.

LOW-GLUCOSE CARBOHYDRATES

Food	Glucose Index	Food	Glucose Index
Nopal, prickly pear cactus	7	Mesquite cake	25
Yogurt, low-fat, unsweetened, plain	14	Kidney beans	27
		Peach, fresh	28
Acorns, stewed, with venison	16	Beans, dried	29
Soybeans	18	Lentils	29
Rice bran	19	Yellow tepary bean broth	29
Cherries	22	Green beans	30
Peas, dried	22	Black beans	30
Plum	24	Apricot, dried	31
Barley	25	Butter beans	31
Grapefruit	25	Skim milk	32

LOW-GLUCOSE CARBOHYDRATES (continued)

Food	Glucose Index	Food	Glucose Index
Lima beans, baby, frozen	32	Pinto beans	39
Split peas, yellow, boiled	32	Corn hominy	40
Chickpeas	33	All Bran	42
Rye rice	34	Black-eyed beans	42
Apple	36	Grapes	43
Pear	36	Orange	43
Spaghetti, whole wheat	37	Spirali, durum	43
Haricot (navy) beans	38	Mixed grain	45
Star pastina, boiled 5 min.	38		
Tomato	38		
Tortilla	38		
Brown beans	38		

Table adapted with permission from the *American Journal of Clinical Nutrition* 62 (1995): 871–935.

B.

MAXIMUM GRAMS OF PROTEIN INTAKE PER DAY

Weight (in pounds)	Level of Activity				
	1	2	3	4	5
100	36g	55g	59g	77g	91g
110	40	60	65	85	100
120	44	65	71	93	109
130	47	71	77	100	118
140	51	76	83	108	127
150	55	82	89	116	136
160	58	87	95	124	145
170	62	93	100	131	155
180	65	98	106	139	164
190	69	104	112	147	173
200	73	109	118	155	182
210	76	115	124	162	191
220	80	120	130	170	200
230	84	125	136	178	209

MAXIMUM GRAMS OF PROTEIN INTAKE PER DAY

Weight (in pounds)	Level of Activity				
	1	2	3	4	5
240	87	131	142	185	218
250	91	136	148	193	227
260	95	142	154	201	236

Step one: Determine your level of physical activity.

Level 1: You are sedentary, do light weight training or less than 40 minutes of aerobics a day.

Level 2: You are a seasoned body builder who trains four days a week.

Level 3: You are a serious aerobic athlete training 60–90 minutes a day.

Level 4: You are just beginning a program of building substantial amounts of muscle and plan to train at least four days a week.

Level 5: You are a professional athlete.

Step two: Determine how many grams of protein you require in a day. First, find your activity level along the top of the table. Follow down that column until you find the number opposite your weight in pounds. That's the maximum grams of protein intake per day for which there is at least some scientific evidence of efficacy.

LEAN PROTEINS

Product	Amount	Calories	Protein (grams)	Fat (grams)	Total Carbos	Excess Nonprotein Calories
Nonfat vanilla yogurt	1 cup	195	12	0	0	0
Protein powder, soy	2 heaping Tbsp	80	18	0	0	0
Protein powder, egg	2 heaping Tbsp	100	24	0	0	0
Egg white	1 large	16	3.4	0	0.6	2
Greenland turbot	3 oz.	74	14.7	0.3		3
Protein powder, milk	2 heaping Tbsp	110	25	0	1	4
Snow crab	3 oz.	84	18.3	0.6		5
Croaker	3 oz.	82	17.9	0.63		6
Lingcod	3 oz.	87	19	0.64		6
Pacific cod	3 oz.	82	17.8	0.67		6
Dolphin	3 oz.	87	19	0.69		6

LEAN PROTEINS (continued)

Product	Amount	Calories	Protein (grams)	Fat (grams)	Total Carbos	Excess Nonprotein Calories
Walleye pike	3 oz.	88	19.3	0.69		6
Cod, baked	3 oz.	89	19.4	0.7	0	6
Eel	3 oz.	85	18.5	0.7		6
Snapper	3 oz.	89	19.6	0.7		6
Halibut	3 oz.	87	18.9	0.72		6
Clams (raw)	3 oz.	105	17.1	0.76		7
Shrimp	3 oz.	88	16.8	0.76		7
Pompano	3 oz.	81	17.2	0.8		7
Carp	3 oz.	90	19.3	0.81		7
Atlantic herring	3 oz.	102	21.9	0.9		8
Spiny lobster	3 oz.	90	18.8	0.9		8
Whitefish	3 oz.	108	23.4	0.95		9
Mahimahi (dolphin fillet)	3 oz.	108	23.4	0.95		9
Blue crab	3 oz.	74	12.8	0.97		9
King crab	3 oz.	86	17.4	0.97		9
Alaskan pollock	3 oz.	92	19.4	0.98		9
Yellowfin tuna	3 oz.	103	22	1.01		9
Haddock	3 oz.	92	19.4	1.02		9
Atlantic mackerel	3 oz.	85	17.7	1.06		10
Northern lobster	3 oz.	89	18.7	1.06		10
Dungeness crab	3 oz.	87	18.1	1.08		10
Hawaiian wahoo	3 oz.	94	19.3	1.1		10
Crayfish	3 oz.	90	18.5	1.18		11
Golden kingklip	3 oz.	91	18.8	1.19		11
Spot	3 oz.	91	18	1.19		11
Rainbow trout	3 oz.	93	19.1	1.22		11
Turbot	3 oz.	90	18.3	1.31		12
Sole	3 oz.	100	20.5	1.34		12
Orange roughy	3 oz.	91	18.5	1.4		13
Mussels (blue)	3 oz.	112	20.6	1.51		14
Mullet	3 oz.	76	14.5	1.52		14
Sablefish	3 oz.	94	18.8	1.57		14
Pacific ocean perch	3 oz.	94	18.6	1.63		15
Butterfish	3 oz.	98	20.7	1.7		15

LEAN PROTEINS

Product	Amount	Calories	Protein (grams)	Fat (grams)	Total Carbos	Excess Nonprotein Calories
Snails (unspec. raw)	3 oz.	106	20.3	1.73		16
Nonfat cottage cheese	1 cup	123	28	0.6	2.7	16
Cusk	3 oz.	94	18.8	1.9		17
Squid	3 oz.	75	14.4	1.9		17
Pacific jack mackerel	3 oz.	105	20.3	2		18
Sea trout	3 oz.	97	18.4	2		18
Tuna, white, canned in water	3 oz.	116	22.7	2.1	0	19
Eastern and Gulf oysters	3 oz.	86	11.9	2.24		20
Bigeye tuna	3 oz.	110	20.8	2.29		21
Scallops	3 oz.	81	9.45	2.3		21
Opakapaka	3 oz.	124	24.1	2.3		21
Albacore tuna	3 oz.	96	17.5	2.31		21
Swordfish	3 oz.	97	17.7	2.33		21
Abalone	3 oz.	98	18.5	2.4		22
Tilapia	3 oz.	97	17.6	2.42		22
Pacific oysters	3 oz.	69	7.06	2.47		22
Atlantic cod	3 oz.	111	20.5	2.5		23
Whey protein — 80%	2 heaping Tbsp	100	20	1.8	2	24
Redfish	3 oz.	105	18.9	2.73		25
Chicken breast, no skin, roasted	3 oz.	142	26.7	3.1	0	28
Crevalle jack	3 oz.	104	17.8	3.17		29
Turkey breast, no skin, roasted	3.5 oz.	157	29.9	3.2	0	29
Shad, baked	3 oz.	118	20.6	3.36		30
Venison, lean, raw	3 oz.	107	17.9	3.4	0	31
Sockeye salmon	3 oz.	116	19.9	3.45		31
Grouper	3 oz.	99	16.9	3.5		32
Atlantic ocean perch	3 oz.	103	17.6	3.6		32

LEAN PROTEINS (continued)

Product	Amount	Calories	Protein (grams)	Fat (grams)	Total Carbos	Excess Nonprotein Calories
Shad	3 oz.	104	16.7	3.61		32
Ocean catfish	3 oz.	117	19.4	3.79		34
Tilefish	3 oz.	121	19.8	4.01		36
Blue runner	3 oz.	124	20	4.24		38
Lake trout	3 oz.	116	18.2	4.26		38
Skate (ray)	3 oz.	130	21	4.51		41
Pork tenderloin, trimmed, roasted	3.5 oz.	166	28.8	4.8	0	43
Rockfish	3 oz.	117	18.5	4.8		43
Bluefish	3 oz.	131	20.4	4.84		44
Reduced-fat cheese	1 oz.	73	6	4.5	0.8	44
Skipjack tuna	3 oz.	144	23.3	4.9		44
Striped bass	3 oz.	123	18.5	4.9		44
Yeast, dry baker's	1 oz.	80	10.5	0.5	11	49
Skim milk	1 cup	86	8	0.2	11.9	49
Catfish (channel)	3 oz.	127	17.8	5.6		50
Whiting	3 oz.	134	19.1	5.86		53
Egg, whole (chicken)	1 large	79	6.1	5.6	0.6	53
Pink salmon	3 oz.	146	21.6	5.95		54
Round steak, trimmed, broiled	3.5 oz.	191	31.7	6.2	0	56
Salmon, canned	3 oz.	130	17.4	6.2	0	56
Monkfish	3 oz.	139	19.3	6.3		57
Mozzarella cheese	1 oz.	80	7	6.1	0.6	57
Lake whitefish	3 oz.	148	20.8	6.61		59
Atlantic pollock	3 oz.	126	14.7	7		63
Northern pike	3 oz.	140	18.5	7.2		65
Buttermilk	1 cup	99	8	2.2	11.7	67
Bluefin tuna	3 oz.	177	25.3	7.6		68
Parmesan cheese	1 oz.	111	10	7.3	0.9	69
1% milk	1 cup	102	8	2.4	12.2	70
Provolone cheese	1 oz.	100	7	7.6	0.6	71
Spanish mackerel	3 oz.	157	20.1	7.89		71
Bonito	3 oz.	145	17.3	8.02		72
Cottage cheese, 2% fat	1 cup	203	31.1	4.4	8.2	72

LEAN PROTEINS

Product	Amount	Calories	Protein (grams)	Fat (grams)	Total Carbos	Excess Nonprotein Calories
Gouda cheese	1 oz.	101	7	7.8	0.6	73
Yogurt, plain nonfat	1 cup	140	14	0.4	17.4	73
Flounder, baked	3.5 oz.	202	30	8.2	0	74
Yogurt, nonfat frozen	½ cup	100	4	0.1	18.7	76
Atlantic sardines, canned, in oil	3 oz.	168	21.3	8.56		77
Monterey Jack cheese	1 oz.	106	8	8.6	0.2	78
Pacific herring	3 oz.	158	18	9.04		81
Porgy	3 oz.	164	18.5	9.47		85
Coho salmon	3 oz.	180	20.1	10.44		94
Yogurt, low-fat plain	1 cup	159	13	3.5	16	96
Pacific sardines, canned in tomato sauce	3 oz.	208	24.6	11.46		103
Flounder	3 oz.	184	18.4	11.66		105
Yogurt, low-fat frozen	½ cup	110	4	3.5	18.7	106
Sea bass	3 oz.	178	16.4	11.98		108
Part-skim ricotta cheese	½ cup	171	14	9.8	6.4	114
Smelt	3 oz.	197	16.9	13.77		124
Shark	3 oz.	197	16.9	13.77		124
Ling	3 oz.	195	16.4	13.88		125
King mackerel	3 oz.	205	18.6	13.89		125
Chocolate (1% fat) milk	1 cup	158	8	2.5	26.1	127
Chinook salmon	3 oz.	195	13.4	15.3		138
Ground beef, extra lean, baked	3.5 oz.	274	30.3	16	0	144
Yogurt, low-fat vanilla	1 cup	209	12	2.8	31.3	150
American cheese	2 oz. (slices)	212	12.6	17.8	1	164
Peanut butter, smooth	2 Tbsp	188	9	16	5.4	166

LEAN PROTEINS (continued)

Product	Amount	Calories	Protein (grams)	Fat (grams)	Total Carbos	Excess Nonprotein Calories
Yogurt, low-fat fruit-flavored	1 cup	227	10	2.6	42.3	193
Big Mac hamburger	1 burger	570	24.6	35	39.2	472

C.

OMEGA-3 FATTY ACIDS IN FISH AND FISH OILS

Fish Oils/Fish	Omega-3 Fatty Acids		Total Fish Oil (per 100 grams)
	EPA	DHA	
MaxEPATM, concentrated fish body oils	17.8	11.6	29.4
Menhaden oil	12.7	7.9	20.6
Salmon oil	8.8	11.1	19.9
Cod liver oil	9.0	9.5	18.5
Herring oil	7.1	4.3	11.4
Atlantic mackerel	0.9	1.6	2.5
King mackerel	1	1.2	2.2
Muroaji scad	0.5	1.5	2.0
Chub mackerel	0.9	1	1.9
Spiny dogfish	0.7	1.2	1.9
Japanese horse mackerel	0.5	1.3	1.8
Pacific herring	1.0	0.7	1.7
Atlantic herring	0.7	0.9	1.6
Lake trout	0.5	1.1	1.6
Bluefin tuna	0.4	1.2	1.6
Atlantic sturgeon	1.0	0.5	1.5
Sablefish	0.7	0.7	1.4
Chinook salmon	0.8	0.6	1.4
European anchovy	0.5	0.9	1.4
Albacore tuna	0.3	1.0	1.3
Lake whitefish	0.3	1.0	1.3
Saury	0.5	0.8	1.3
European sole	0.5	0.8	1.3
Sprat	0.5	0.8	1.3
Atlantic salmon	0.3	0.9	1.2
Round herring	0.4	0.8	1.2
Sockeye salmon	0.5	0.7	1.2
Bluefish	0.4	0.8	1.2

OMEGA-3 FATTY ACIDS IN FISH AND FISH OILS

Fish Oils/Fish	Omega-3 Fatty Acids		Total Fish Oil (per 100 grams)
	EPA	DHA	
Unspecified mullet	0.5	0.6	1.1
Chum salmon	0.4	0.6	1.0
Coho salmon	0.3	0.5	0.8
Pink salmon	0.4	0.6	1.0
Unspecified conch	0.6	0.4	1.0
Greenland halibut	0.5	0.4	0.9
Striped bass	0.2	0.6	0.8
Rainbow smelt	0.3	0.4	0.7
Rockfish	0.3	0.4	0.7
Pompano	0.2	0.4	0.6
Pacific oyster	0.4	0.2	0.6
Horse mackerel	0.3	0.3	0.6
Swordfish	0.1	0.5	0.6
Arctic char trout	0.1	0.5	0.6
Atlantic wolffish	0.3	0.3	0.6
Common periwinkle	0.5	0	0.5
Freshwater drum	0.2	0.3	0.5
Silver hake	0.2	0.3	0.5
Striped mullet	0.3	0.2	0.5
Rainbow trout	0.1	0.4	0.5
European oyster	0.3	0.2	0.5
Pacific hake	0.2	0.3	0.5
Pollock	0.1	0.4	0.5
Canary rockfish	0.2	0.3	0.5
Unspecified rockfish	0.2	0.3	0.5
Unspecified shark	0	0.5	0.5
Unspecified tuna	0.1	0.4	0.5
Japanese (kuruma) prawn	0.3	0.2	0.5
Northern shrimp	0.3	0.2	0.5
Blue mussel	0.2	0.3	0.5
Brook trout	0.2	0.2	0.4
Brown bullhead catfish	0.2	0.2	0.4
Cisco	0.1	0.3	0.4
Pacific halibut	0.1	0.3	0.4
Carp	0.2	0.1	0.3
Sweet smelt	0.2	0.1	0.3
European eel	0.1	0.1	0.2

U.S. Department of Agriculture

Part One.
"Maximize Alertness:
Problem Solving"

To find out whether you're a morning or an evening person, a lark or an owl, take J. A. Horne's and O. Oestberg's test printed below. Once you've scored the test and discovered your type, return to the "Problem Solving" chapter for further advice on how best to use your "morningness" or "eveningness."

OWL AND LARK QUESTIONNAIRE
By J. A. Horne and O. Oestberg

Instructions:

1. Please read each question very carefully before answering.
2. Answer ALL questions.
3. Answer questions in numerical order.
4. Each question should be answered independently of others. Do NOT go back and check your answers.
5. All questions have a selection of answers. For each question place a cross alongside ONE answer only. Some questions have a scale instead of a selection of answers. Place a cross at the appropriate point along the scale.

1. Considering only your own "feeling best" rhythm, at what time would you get up if you were entirely free to plan your day?

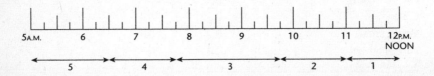

2. Considering only your own "feeling best" rhythm, at what time would you go to bed if you you were entirely free to plan your evening?

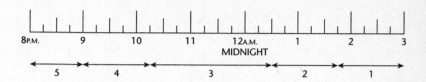

3. If there is a specific time at which you have to get up in the morning, to what extent are you dependent on being woken up by an alarm clock?

Not at all dependent   ❏ 4

Slightly dependent   ❏ 3

Fairly dependent   ❏ 2

Very dependent   ❏ 1

4. Assuming adequate environmental conditions, how easy do you find getting up in the mornings?

Not at all easy   ❏ 1

Not very easy   ❏ 2

Fairly easy   ❏ 3

Very easy   ❏ 4

5. How alert do you feel during the first half-hour after having woken in the mornings?

Not at all alert   ❏ 1

Slightly alert   ❏ 2

Fairly alert   ❏ 3

Very alert   ❏ 4

6. How is your appetite during the first half-hour after having awoken in the mornings?

Very poor	❑ 1
Fairly poor	❑ 2
Fairly good	❑ 3
Very good	❑ 4

7. During the first half-hour after having woken in the morning, how tired do you feel?

Very tired	❑ 1
Fairly tired	❑ 2
Fairly refreshed	❑ 3
Very refreshed	❑ 4

8. When you have no commitments the next day, at what time do you go to bed compared to your usual bedtime?

Seldom or never later	❑ 4
Less than an hour later	❑ 3
1–2 hours later	❑ 2
More than 2 hours later	❑ 1

9. You have decided to engage in some physical exercise. A friend suggests that you do this one hour twice a week and the best time for him is between 7:00 and 8:00 A.M. Bearing in mind nothing else but your own "feeling best" rhythm, how do you think you would perform?

Would be in good form	❑ 4
Would be in reasonable form	❑ 3
Would find it difficult	❑ 2
Would find it very difficult	❑ 1

10. At what time in the evening do you feel tired and as a result in need of sleep?

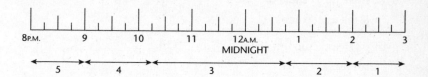

11. You wish to be at your peak performance for a test which you know is going to be mentally exhausting and lasting for two hours. You are entirely free to plan your day and considering only your own "feeling best" rhythm, which ONE of the four testing times would you choose?

8:00–10:00 A.M.	❏ 6
11:00 A.M.–1:00 P.M.	❏ 4
3:00–5:00 P.M.	❏ 2
7:00–9:00 P.M.	❏ 0

12. If you went to bed at 11:00 P.M. at what level of tiredness would you be?

Not at all tired	❏ 0
A little tired	❏ 2
Fairly tired	❏ 3
Very tired	❏ 5

13. For some reason you have gone to bed several hours later than usual, but there is no need to get up at any particular time the next morning. Which ONE of the following events are you most likely to experience?

Will wake up at usual time and will NOT fall asleep	❏ 4

Will wake up at the usual time   ❑ 3
    and will doze thereafter

Will wake up at usual time but   ❑ 2
    will fall asleep again

Will NOT wake up until later   ❑ 1
    than usual

14. One night you have to remain awake between 4:00 and 6:00 A.M. in order to carry out a night watch. You have no commitments the next day. Which ONE of the following alternatives will suit you best?

Would NOT go to bed until   ❑ 1
    watch was over

Would take a nap before   ❑ 2
    and sleep after

Would take a good sleep before   ❑ 3
    and nap after

Would take ALL sleep before watch   ❑ 4

15. You have to do two hours of hard physical work. You are entirely free to plan your day and considering only your own "feeling best" rhythm, which ONE of the following times would you choose?

8:00–10:00 A.M.   ❑ 4

11:00 A.M.–1:00 P.M.   ❑ 3

3:00–5:00 P.M.   ❑ 2

7:00–9:00 P.M.   ❑ 1

16. You have decided to engage in hard physical exercise. A friend suggests that you do this for one hour twice a week and the best time for him is between 10:00 and 11:00 P.M. Bearing in mind nothing else but your

own "feeling best" rhythm, how well do you think you would perform?

Would be in good form ❑ 1

Would be in reasonable form ❑ 2

Would find it difficult ❑ 3

Would find it very difficult ❑ 4

17. Suppose that you can choose your own work hours. Assume that you worked a FIVE-hour day (including breaks) and that your job was interesting and paid by results. Which FIVE CONSECUTIVE HOURS would you select?

12 1 2 3 4 5 6 7 8 9 10 11 12 1 2 3 4 5 6 7 8 9 10 11 12
MIDNIGHT   NOON   MIDNIGHT

1   5   4   3   2   1

18. At what time of the day do you think that you reach your "feeling best" peak?

12 1 2 3 4 5 6 7 8 9 10 11 12 1 2 3 4 5 6 7 8 9 10 11 12
MIDNIGHT   NOON   MIDNIGHT

1   5   4   3   2   1

19. One hears about "morning" and "evening" types of people. Which ONE of these types do you consider your-self to be?

Definitely a "morning" type ❑ 6

Rather more a "morning" than
   an "evening" type ❑ 4

Rather more an "evening" than a
   "morning" type ❑ 2

Definitely an "evening" type ❑ 0

Scoring:

- For questions 3, 4, 5, 6, 7, 8, 9, 11, 12, 13, 14, 15, 16, and 19, note for each response the appropriate score displayed beside the answer box.

- For questions 1, 2, 10, and 18, refer the cross made along each scale to the appropriate score value range below the scale.

- For question 17 take the most extreme cross on the right-hand side as the reference point and take the appropriate score value range below this point.

- Add together the scores and convert the sum into a five-point Morningness–Eveningness scale:

Score	
Definitely Morning Type	70–86
Moderately Morning Type	59–69
Neither Type	42–58
Moderately Evening Type	31–41
Definitely Evening Type	16–30

Part Two.
"Step 3: Play to
Your Strengths"

Look below for the personality that matches the four-letter score you received after taking the test in the Step "Play to Your Strengths." Jonathan Niednagel, Director of the Brain Type Institute in California, has prepared these "personality profiles" especially for this book. There are two broad divisions, introverts and extroverts. Within each personality type you will find the following descriptions.

1. Popular Career Choices: These are careers that people who share this personality type are most likely to choose.
2. What is important to know about this type at work: Here you'll find the inborn skills of people with this personality type as well as their desired work environment.
3. Best approach to this personality type: This is key to the Step "Practice Emotional Broadcasting." If you're going to connect with someone, here's what you need to know about them.
4. People who may share this personality profile: These are famous or successful people who may have this personality type.

Introverts

The following eight brain types are introverts. The single feature which distinguishes an introvert best is a preference for drawing energy from one's internal world of ideas, emotions, or impressions instead of drawing that energy from others. Introverts are energy conservers; the adjective for introverts is "fewer," that is fewer friends, fewer projects, etc. Introverts do not show as much eye contact when they're speaking, although they might show as much eye contact as extroverts when they're listening. Here are the other adjectives and qualities attributed to introverts:

- inner world
- reflective
- energy conserving
- reserved
- defensive
- private
- needs time to express himself or herself
- meditative
- softer voice

ISFP

"ARTISAN"

Overview: Appreciates beauty and texture; artistic, athletic, and graceful; reticent, not verbally expressive; realistic; sensitive, modest, kind; sympathetic; impulsive, enjoys freedom; service-oriented; gross motor skilled

1. At which vocations would an ISFP be best?

   Popular career choices:

   Artist, dancer, athlete, musician, photographer, fashion designer, child-care worker, nurse, animal-care specialist, minister, transportation operative, construction worker, farmer

2. What is important to know about an ISFP at work:

   Inborn skills: introspective/thorough, pragmatic, caring, adaptable

   Desired work environment: calm, practical, friendly, flexible

   Common job descriptions: artist, photographer, care-giver, athlete

3. Best approach to this personality type:

needs someone who is a good listener, not pushy, down-to-
earth, affectionate, complimentary, sympathetic, loyal,
appreciative, tolerant

4. People who may share this personality profile:

Alan Jackson   Janet Jackson

Michael Johnson   Jackie Joyner-Kersee

Mark McGwire   Kathy Whitworth

Scottie Pippen

Bill "Willie" Shoemaker

Chuck Yeager

ISFJ

"ASSISTANT"

Overview: concerned with others' welfare; responsible, reserved,
patient, practical, friendly, orderly, inquisitive regarding people,
harm-avoiding; conscientious, thorough, loyal; service-oriented;
gross motor skilled

1. At which vocations would an ISFJ be best?

Popular career choices:

Nursing, social service work, ministry, secretarial service,
teaching (especially elementary level), counseling, child
care, probation work, veterinary medicine, physical
therapy

2. What is important to know about an ISFJ at work:

Inborn skills: introspective/thorough, pragmatic, caring,
organized

Desired work environment: calm, practical, friendly,
structured

Common job descriptions: assistant, social worker, nurse

3. Best approach to this personality type:

needs someone who is a good listener, not pushy, well-groomed, affectionate, empathetic, complimentary, loyal/responsible, appreciative

4. People who may share this personality profile:

This type is not found in the limelight, except in professional sports.

Richmond Webb (All-Pro NFL tackle)

Walter Ray Williams Jr. (bowler)

NBA players:

P. J. Brown

A. C. Earl

Andrew Lang

Alton Lister

ISTP

"ATHLETE"

Overview: Artful with machines, tools, and hands; seeks action and excitement; superb tactician — seizing the moment; athletic, competitive; witty but usually not wordy; street smart; ever-thinking; can be intense with deep convictions; adaptive; fine motor skilled

1. At which vocations would an ISTP be best?

Popular career choices:

Construction, mechanics, machine operation, racing, aviation, surgery, sculpting, securities trading, finance, law enforcement, criminal investigation, the masters of tools and machines

2. What is important to know about an ISTP at work:

Inborn skills: introspective/thorough, pragmatic, logical, adaptable

Desired work environment: calm, practical, rational, flexible

Common job descriptions: artisan, athlete, law enforcement officer

3. Best approach to this personality type:

needs someone who is a good listener, down-to-earth, interested in thought, not too emotional, flexible

4. People who may share this personality profile:

Larry Bird	Bonnie Blair
Roger Clemens	Steffi Graf
Mike Ditka	Martina Navratilova
Michael Jordan	Monica Seles
Carl Karcher	Mary Decker Slancy
John McEnroe	
General Norman Schwarzkopf	
Mike Tyson	

ISTJ

"INVESTIGATOR"

Overview: gatherer of data; compelled to identify reality and bring order; stable, conservative, dependable, reserved, logical, fastidious, systematic, painstaking, thorough, dutiful; fine motor skilled

1. At which vocations would an ISTJ be best?

Popular career choices:

Law, legal secretary, dentistry, banking, accounting, tax examining, financial planning, insurance, teaching, coaching, engineering, computer programming, physical sciences, supervising or managing, law enforcement, military, fire fighting, farming

2. What is important to know about an ISTJ at work:

   Inborn skills: introspective/thorough, pragmatic, logical, organized

   Desired work environment: calm, practical, rational, structured

   Common job descriptions: investigator, auditor

3. Best approach to this personality type:

   needs someone who is a good listener, not pushy, well groomed, loyal/responsible, trustworthy, appreciative, has convictions

4. People who may share this personality profile:

Tom Landry	Queen Elizabeth II
Jack Nicklaus	Chris Evert Lloyd
Alan Simpson	Pat Nixon
John Wooden	

INFP

"IDEALIST"

Overview: deep internal values; idealistic, romantic, appears calm; generally reticent; creative, avoids conflict, sensitive, aware of others' feelings; sacrificial, welcomes new ideas; flexible, interested in learning and writing; composer; language skilled

1. At which vocations would an INFP be best?

   Popular career choices:

   Psychology, psychiatry, medicine, science, teaching (prefer higher levels of education), counseling, religious education, ministry and missionary work, literature, art, music, composing and writing, poetry

2. What is important to know about an INFP at work:

    Inborn skills: introspective/thorough, imaginative, caring, adaptable

    Desired work environment: calm, creative, friendly, flexible

    Common job descriptions: composer, poet, counselor

3. Best approach to this personality type:

    needs someone who is a good listener, not pushy, harmonious, affectionate, complimentary, romantic, loyal, understanding, appreciative, tolerant

4. People who may share this personality profile:

    Julius Erving (Dr. J)   Mother Teresa

    Jim Henson

    Michael Jackson

    Christian Riese Lassen

    Charles Schulz

    James Taylor

INFJ

"WORDSMITH"

Overview: Potential as gifted writer; imaginative, conscientious; has concern for the needs and development of others; empathetic; enjoys enriching inner life; methodical; quietly forceful; counselor; language skilled

1. At which vocations would an INFJ be best?

    Popular career choices:

    Psychology, psychiatry, therapy, counseling, ministry, religious educator, scientific research, medicine, journalism, writing and editing, teaching

2. What is important to know about an INFJ at work:

Inborn skills: introspective/thorough, imaginative, caring, organized

Desired work environment: calm, creative, friendly, structured

Common job descriptions: writer, counselor, physician

3. Best approach to this personality type:

needs someone who is reflective, affectionate, complimentary, romantic, loyal, values the meaningful, seeks to develop self and others

4. People who may share this personality profile:

Lamar Hunt

William Phillips (book editor)

Leigh Steinberg (sports agent)

INTP

"LOGICIAN"

Overview: master of conceptual logic; problem-solver; scientific — desires understanding of universe; designs logical models; seeks precision; introspective; adaptable; tends to excel in theoretical, philosophical subjects; skilled at logical abstraction

1. At which vocations would an INTP be best?

Popular career choices:

Mathematics, philosophy, psychiatry, medicine, advanced sciences, university teaching, physics, scientific research, strategic planning, creative writing, literature, music, art

2. What is important to know about an INTP at work:

Inborn skills: introspective/thorough, imaginative, logical, adaptable

Desired work environment: calm, creative, competent, flexible

Common job descriptions: scientist/researcher, philosopher

3. Best approach to this personality type:

needs someone who is reflective, flexible, interested in deep thought and meaning, considers rational possibilities

4. People who may share this personality profile:

Arthur Ashe   Mary-Jo Fernandez

William F. Buckley Jr.   Jane Goodall

George Washington Carver

Leonardo da Vinci

Albert Einstein

John Lennon

Nelson Mandela

Steven Spielberg

INTJ

"INVENTOR"

Overview: applicator of ideas; builder of theoretical systems; self-confident; independent, reserved, single-minded, conceptual; seeks knowledge; not impressed with authority; determined, analytic, stubborn, skeptical, scientific; skilled at logical abstraction

1. At which vocations would an INTJ be best?

Popular career choices:

Engineering, inventing, computer science, law, consulting, management, research, medicine, science (life and physical), languages, entrepreneur, business analyst, and careers involving the management of human resources

2. What is important to know about an INTJ at work:

Inborn skills: introspective/thorough, imaginative, logical, organized

Desired work environment: calm, creative, competent, structure

Common job descriptions: inventor, engineer, lawyer, analyst

3. Best approach to this personality type:

someone who is a good listener, reflective, values the meaningful; appreciates analysis, logic, and intelligence; has convictions

4. People who may share this personality profile:

Warren Beatty	Justice Ruth Ginsburg
Jimmy Carter	Nancy Kassebaum
Prince Charles	Justice Sandra Day O'Connor
Abraham Lincoln	
Ralph Nader	

Extroverts

These following eight brain types are extroverts. Extroverts are energized by the external world, the world around them. Their preference is for drawing energy from the outside world of people, places, activities, or things. Extroverts are energy expenders; the adjective for extroverts is "many," that is many friends, many projects, many things going on. Here are the other adjectives and qualities attributed to extroverts:

• outer world

• active

• energy expending

• expressive

- aggressive
- expanding
- public
- reasons out loud
- louder voice

ESFP

"ENTERTAINER"

Overview: performs to entertain others; enjoys creating party-like atmosphere; spender—not a saver; expressive; down-to-earth; radiates warmth and optimism; impulsive, enjoys promoting and business; rhythmical and athletic; gross motor skilled

1. At which vocations would an ESFP be best?

   Popular career choices:

   Tour and travel, sales, public relations, catering, performing arts, athletics, nursing, child care, cosmetology, designing, transportation operatives, construction

2. What is important to know about an ESFP at work:

   Inborn skills: energetic, pragmatic, caring, adaptable

   Desired work environment: active, practical, friendly, flexible

   Common job descriptions: adjuster, entertainer, travel agent, promoter

3. Best approach to this personality type:

   needs someone who is attentive, down-to-earth, affectionate, complimentary, sympathetic, a hugger, loyal, fun-loving/enjoys life, appreciative, tolerant

4. People who may share this personality profile:

Muhammad Ali   Sarah Brightman

Ken Griffey Jr.   Aretha Franklin

Magic Johnson   Florence Griffith Joyner

Carl Lewis   Dolly Parton

Elvis Presley   Ivana Trump

ESFJ

"FACILITATOR"

Overview: hospitable, focuses on usefulness; energetic, realistic; develops and nurtures relationships; sensitive to praise and criticism; expresses feelings; conscientious; orderly; friendly promoter, commerce-oriented; gross motor skilled

1. At which vocations would an ESFJ be best?

   Popular career choices:

   Sales, customer relations, business, residential real estate, supervisor, secretary, teaching (especially elementary level), special education, ministry, nursing, psychology, social work; in general, jobs where contact with people is involved

2. What is important to know about an ESFJ at work:

   Inborn skills: energetic, pragmatic, caring, organized

   Desired work environment: active, practical, friendly, structured

   Common job descriptions: customer relations representative, salesperson, counselor, facilitator

3. Best approach to this personality type:

   needs someone who is attentive, well groomed, affectionate, complimentary, empathetic, sentimental, a hugger, loyal/responsible, appreciative, has a sense of reality

4. People who may share this personality profile:

Family advocates: Barbara Bush

   Dr. James Dobson   Princess Diana

   Gary Smalley   Queen Mother Elizabeth
                                  (former Lady Elizabeth
                                  Bowes-Lyon)

                        Tipper Gore

                        Nancy Kerrigan

                        Loretta Lynn

ESTJ

"SUPERVISOR"

Overview: excels at organizing and running activities and orderly procedures; matter-of-fact; consistent, efficient, energetic, pragmatic, critiquing; likes rules and laws; values traditions; commerce-oriented; fine motor skilled

1. At which vocations would an ESTJ be best?

   Popular career choices:

   Employment that involves money, facts, and objects: business, management, finance, banking, commerce, accounting, law, home economics, teaching, school administration, cosmetology, secretarial, law enforcement, military

2. What is important to know about an ESTJ at work:

   Inborn skills: energetic, pragmatic, logical, organized

   Desired work environment: active, practical, rational, structured

   Common job descriptions: administrator, supervisor, manager

3. Best approach to this personality type:

 needs someone who is attentive, well groomed, loyal/
 responsible, trustworthy, appreciative, values logic

4. People who may share this personality profile:

 Bob Dole   Geraldine Ferraro

 Gerald Ford   Rose Kennedy

 Richard Nixon

 Nolan Ryan

 Harry Truman

ESTP

"OPPORTUNIST"

Overview: "smooth operator," deal-maker; tactical, enterprising;
adaptable, persuasive, energetic; seeks fun and excitement; athletic;
enjoys the moment; realistic, good-natured, self-focused; body- and
clothes-conscious; entrepreneur; negotiator; promoter; fine motor
skilled

1. At which vocations would an ESTP be best?

 Popular career choices:

 Sales, real estate, investments, entrepreneur, automobile
 dealer, mechanic, athletics, dentistry, construction, multi-
 level marketing

2. What is important to know about an ESTP at work:

 Inborn skills: energetic, pragmatic, logical, adaptable

 Desired work environment: active, practical, rational, flexible

 Common job descriptions: promoter, athlete, salesperson

3. Best approach to this personality type:

 needs someone who is attentive, observant, tolerant,
 flexible, uses common sense, enjoys life/fun-loving

4. People who may share this personality profile:

Hulk Hogan   Kim Basinger

Lee Iococca   Cher

Lyndon B. Johnson   Sarah Ferguson (Duchess of York)

Mickey Mantle   Madonna

Joe Montana   Lorrie Morgan

Joe Namath   Tina Turner

Arnold Palmer

Arnold Schwarzenegger

Sylvester Stallone

John Wayne

ENFP

"MOTIVATOR"

Overview: highly energetic; enthusiastic, charming, imaginative, improvisational; sees possibilities; spontaneous; easily bored with repetition; enjoys solving people's problems; catalyst, marketer; language skilled

1. At which vocations would an ENFP be best?

   Popular career choices:

   Sales, public relations, entrepreneur, human services, health-related professions, music, acting and entertaining, play and screen writing, journalism, advertising, ministry, counseling, psychology (note the great latitude in career choices)

2. What is important to know about an ENFP at work:

   Inborn skills: energetic, imaginative, caring, adaptable

   Desired work environment: active, creative, friendly, flexible

   Common job descriptions: motivator, salesperson, musician

3. Best approach to this personality type:

needs someone who is a dreamer, harmonious, affectionate, complimentary, romantic, loyal, appreciative,
tolerant, seeks harmony and the meaningful

4. People who may share this personality profile:

Fred Astaire	Carol Burnett
Sammy Davis Jr.	Goldie Hawn
Evander Holyfield	Whitney Houston
Bob Hope	Diana Ross
Congressman J. C. Watts	Oprah Winfrey

ENFJ

"EDUCATOR"

Overview: teacher/pastor; socially sophisticated; expressive, ambitious, catalyst, cooperative, devoted, fluent, imaginative, emotional;
opinionated; interested in ideas and possibilities; seeks order; skilled
at language

1. At which vocations would an ENFJ be best?

Popular career choices:

teaching, counseling, psychology, ministry, news media,
advertising, acting, writing, photography, health-related
professions, sales, business, coaching

2. What is important to know about an ENFJ at work:

Inborn skills: energetic, imaginative, caring, organized

Desired work environment: active, creative, friendly,
structured

Common job descriptions: educator, communicator,
pastor

3. Best approach to this personality type:

   needs someone who is attentive, affectionate, complimentary, romantic, loyal, goal-oriented, values the meaningful, seeks to develop self and others

4. People who may share this personality profile:

   George Bush   Cindy Crawford

   Tom Cruise   Elizabeth Dole

   Reverend Billy Graham   Jacqueline Kennedy

   Paul McCartney   Julia Roberts

   Christopher Reeve   Elizabeth Taylor

ENTP

"STRATEGIZER"

Overview: "precocious planner," imaginative, alert to possibilities; quick thinking; likes complexity, computer proficient; enjoys one-upmanship; enthusiastic, outspoken, artistic, comedic, manipulative, spontaneous, entrepreneurial; skilled at logical abstraction

1. At which vocations would an ENTP be best?

   Popular career choices:

   Computers, strategic planning, law, politics, medicine, science, business management, entrepreneur, comedy, magic, sales, inventing, venture capitalism, art, music, school administration, teaching, languages, journalism, coaching

2. What is important to know about an ENTP at work:

   Inborn skills: energetic, imaginative, logical, adaptable

   Desired work environment: active, creative, competent, flexible

   Common job descriptions: actor, entrepreneur, strategist

3. Best approach to this personality type:

   needs someone who is attentive, flexible, appreciates ratio-nal possibilities, has a positive outlook, understands emotion, appreciates creativity

4. People who may share this personality profile:

   Winston Churchill   Whoopi Goldberg

   Bill Cosby   Shirley MacLaine

   Benjamin Franklin   Bette Midler

   Bill Gates   Joan Rivers

   Reverend Jesse Jackson   Barbra Streisand

   Mick Jagger

   Edward Kennedy

   Jay Leno

ENTJ

"CHIEF EXECUTIVE OFFICER"

Overview: born "CEO," driven, takes charge; harnesses people to a distant goal; strategic; expressive; potential good debater and public speaker; seeks vision and purpose; political; self-focused; structured; logical abstraction skilled

1. At which vocations would an ENTJ be best?

   Popular career choices:

   ENTJs have the drive and intellectual aptitude to excel in virtually all vocations, yet they seem to derive their greatest satisfaction from jobs that allow them to exercise their abstract logic while leading and inspiring others. Some of these careers include: law, management in business or industry, educational administration, politics, sales, medicine, entrepreneurial endeavors, financial planning, banking, ministry, consulting, public speaking, writing, organization executive, coaching

2. What is important to know about an ENTJ at work:

Inborn skills: energetic, imaginative, logical, organized

Desired work environment: active, creative, competent, structure

Common job descriptions: chief executive officer (CEO), politician, lawyer

3. Best approach to this personality type:

Needs someone who will listen, see possibilities, appreciate intelligence, has a sense of conviction, is goal-oriented. The softball emotional approach probably isn't going to work here. The ENTJ is looking for a clear prescient view. There's much less of an emotional connection, which is why many bosses are seen as cold-hearted.

4. People who may share this personality profile:

Dwight D. Eisenhower	Lucille Ball
John F. Kennedy	Hillary Clinton
Martin Luther King Jr.	Demi Moore
Ronald Reagan	Margaret Thatcher
Franklin Delano Roosevelt	Barbara Walters

Select Bibliography

Benson, Herbert, with Marg Stark. *Timeless Healing.* New York: Fireside/ Simon and Schuster, 1996.

Berger, Bonnie G., and David R. Owen. "Mood Alteration with Yoga and Swimming: Aerobic Exercise May Not Be Necessary." *Perceptual and Motor Skills* 75 (1992): 1331–1343.

Byrne, A., and D. G. Byrne. "The Effect of Exercise on Depression, Anxiety and Other Mood States: A Review." *Journal of Psychosomatic Research* 37, no. 6 (1993): 565–574.

Damasio, Antonio R. *Descartes' Error.* New York: Grosset/Putnam Books, 1994.

Davidson, Richard J., and Steven K. Sutton. "Affective Neuroscience: The Emergence of a Discipline." *Current Opinion in Neurobiology* 5 (1995): 217–224.

Dijk, Derk-Jan, and Charles A. Czeisler. "Contribution of the Circadian Pacemaker and the Sleep Homeostat to Sleep Propensity, Sleep Structure, Electroencephalographic Slow Waves, and Sleep Spindle Activity in Humans." *Journal of Neuroscience* 15 (May 1995): 3526–3538.

———. "Paradoxical Timing of the Circadian Rhythm of Sleep Propensity Serves to Consolidate Sleep and Wakefulness in Humans." *Neuroscience Letters* 166 (1994): 63–68.

Dunn, Andrea L., Bess H. Marcus, James B. Kampert, Melissa Garcia, Harold W. Kohl, and Steven Blair. "Reduction in Cardiovascular Disease Risk Factors: 6-Month Results from Project *Active.*" *Preventive Medicine* 26 (1997): 883–892.

Flusser, Alan. *Style and the Man.* New York: HarperCollins, 1996.

Gardner, Howard. *Leading Minds.* New York: Basic Books, 1995.

Glasser, William. *Choice Theory.* New York: HarperCollins, 1998.

Hanin, Yuri L. "Emotions and Athletic Performance: Individual Zones of Optimal Functioning Model." *European Yearbook of Sport Psychology* 1 (1997): 29–72.

Hanin, Yuri L., and Pasi Syrjä. "Predicted, Actual, and Recalled Affect in Olympic-Level Soccer Players: Idiographic Assessments on Individualized Scales." *Journal of Sport and Exercise Psychology* 18 (1996): 325–335.

Harte, Jane L., and Georg H. Eifert. "The Effects of Running, Environment, and Attentional Focus on Athletes' Catecholamine and Cortisol Levels and Mood." *Psychophysiology* 32 (1995): 49–54.

Irwin, William, Richard J. Davidson, Mark J. Lowe, Bryan J. Mock, James A. Sorenson, and Patrick A. Turski. "Human Amygdala Activation Detected with Echo-Planar Functional Magnetic Resonance Imaging." *NeuroReport* 7 (1996): 1765–1769.

Jourdain, Robert. *Music, the Brain, and Ecstasy.* New York: Avon Books, 1997.

Keirsey, David. *Please Understand Me II.* California: Prometheus Nemesis Book Company, 1998.

LeDoux, Joseph. *The Emotional Brain.* New York: Simon and Schuster, 1996.

Leproult, Rachel, Olivier Van Reeth, Maria M. Byrne, Jeppe Sturis, and Eve Van Cauter. "Sleepiness, Performance, and Neuroendocrine Function during Sleep Deprivation: Effects of Exposure to Bright Light or Exercise." *Journal of Biological Rhythms* 12 (June 1997): 245–258.

Matthews, Dale A., with Connie Clark. *The Faith Factor.* New York: Viking/Penguin Putnam, 1998.

Monk, Timothy H., Daniel J. Buysse, Charles F. Reynolds III, Sarah L. Berga, David B. Jarrett, Amy E. Begley, and David J. Kupfer. "Circadian Rhythms in Human Performance and Mood under Constant Conditions." *Journal of Sleep Research* 6 (1997): 9–18.

Morgan, William, ed. *Physical Activity & Mental Health.* Washington, D.C.: Taylor & Francis, 1997.

Norden, Michael J. *Beyond Prozac.* New York: HarperCollins, 1995.

Padesky, Christine A., with Dennis Greenberger. *Clinician's Guide to Mind over Mood.* New York: Guilford Press, 1995.

Pate, Russell R., et al. "Physical Activity and Public Health: A Recommendation from the Centers for Disease Control and Prevention and the American College of Sports Medicine." *Journal of the American Medical Association* 273 (February 1, 1995): 402–407.

Robertson, Joel, and Tom Monte. *Natural Prozac.* San Francisco: HarperCollins, 1997.

Seligman, Martin E. P. *Learned Optimism.* New York: Knopf, 1991.

Thayer, Robert E. *The Origin of Everyday Moods.* New York: Oxford University Press, 1996.

Vaughan, Susan C. *The Talking Cure.* New York: Grosset/Putnam, 1997.

West, Tom. *In the Mind's Eye.* New York: Prometheus Books, 1997.

Index